Ethics
for Speech-Language Pathologists and Audiologists

An Illust~~ration Casebook~~

**David L. Irwin,
Ph.D., CCC-SLP**
*Professor and Department
Head, Louisiana State
University Health Sciences
Center-Shreveport*

**Mary Pannbacker,
Ph.D., CCC-SLP**
*Professor, Louisiana State
University Health Sciences
Center-Shreveport*

**Thomas W. Powell,
Ph.D., CCC-SLP**
*Professor and Department
Head, Louisiana State
University Health Sciences
Center-Shreveport*

**Gay T. Vekovius,
M.S., CCC-AUD**
*Associate Professor
(retired), Louisiana State
University Health Sciences
Center-Shreveport*

THOMSON
✳
DELMAR LEARNING Australia Canada Mexico Singapore Spain United Kingdom United States

MW

THOMSON

DELMAR LEARNING

Ethics for Speech-Language Pathologists and Audiologists: An Illustrative Casebook
by David Irwin, Mary Pannbacker, Thomas W. Powell, and Gay T. Vekovius

**Vice President,
Health Care Business Unit:**
William Brottmiller

Product Manager:
Molly Belmont

Channel Manager:
Michele McTighe

Director of Learning Solutions:
Matthew Kane

Editorial Assistant:
Angela Doolin

Production Manager:
Barbara A. Bullock

Acquisitions Editor:
Kalen Conerly

Marketing Director:
Jennifer McAvey

Library of Congress Cataloging-in-Publication Data
Ethics for speech-language pathologists and audiologists : an illustrative casebook/David Irwin . . . [et al.].
    p. ; cm.
    Includes bibliographical references and index.
    ISBN 1-4180-0955-5
    1. Speech therapists—Professional ethics. 2. Audiologists—Professional ethics. I. Irwin, David (David L.)
    [DNLM: 1. Speech-Language Pathology—ethics. 2. Audiology—ethics. 3. Codes of Ethics. 4. Decision Making. WL 340.2 E84 2007]
    RC428.5.E84 2007
    174′.9616855—dc22
                                2006015212
ISBN 1418009555

NOTICE TO THE READER

3/26/07

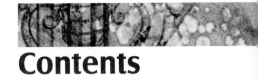

Contents

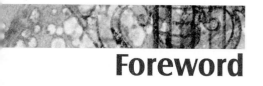

Foreword

Today's clinicians, scholars, and researchers, regardless of where they are in their professional life cycle (student; beginning practitioner; or seasoned, experienced professional), recognize that evolving scopes of practice, technological advances in clinical procedures, and changing arenas for practice all present ethical challenges that generate lively discussion and debate. Conscientious professionals are keenly aware of their responsibility to uphold ethical standards. In doing so, they are eager to discuss and explore current practice issues as they relate to the codes of ethics to which they must adhere.

The academic classroom is where students begin to study issues in professional ethics. What better forum is there for exploring how one's ethical values and beliefs have been and will continue to be shaped? The student of ethics discovers how value differences shaped by religious beliefs, family beliefs, cultural sensitivity, moral teaching, education, and life experiences influence how one approaches professional ethical dilemmas. Ethical predicaments usually involve situations in which the answers are not clear, especially when most professional codes of ethics are broadly written. Often there are legal issues, workplace issues, situational circumstances, and regulatory dictates that impact the situation. The student of ethics discovers that his or her personal worldview of "what is and is not ethical" may not always match the view of the profession, the employer, or an attorney providing legal counsel as to "what is or is not ethical." Through Socratic strategies and questioning techniques, the authors provoke the reader to think about and explore the not so obvious aspects of an issue in order to seek depth of understanding and pursue resolution. Through the skillful use of scenarios, illustrative of a variety of rules found in most codes of ethics, the reader is guided through an analysis and application model for problem solving.

There is no question that this book has application as a lifelong learning tool and a personal reference resource for speech-language pathologists and audiologists. First, the case scenarios familiarize and prepare students early on for the kinds of questions and predicaments they could face in practicum, clinical fellowship, and professional practice situations. Second, professionals when faced with "real-life" issues will find this book—with its content and strategies—a useful reference resource. A very powerful aspect of the book is the presentation of—and opportunity to apply—an ethical decision-making model. The analysis and solution-seeking process suggested can be applied over and over in one's professional life span as a technique for ethical problem solving.

Third, as seasoned professionals take on new projects, new employment, or shifts in professional interests, the book offers review of ethical issues that may be relevant to different work settings or new professional responsibilities. Finally, as professionals engage in continuing education, this book will serve as an excellent basis for employee professional development, a professional study group activity, or other activities that may satisfy requirements for certification maintenance. This is truly a text in applied ethics.

Nancy P. Huffman, CCC-AUD/SLP
Former Chair, ASHA Board of Ethics

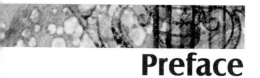

Preface

Introduction

This book is intended for audiology and speech-language pathology students as well as practicing professionals who wish to learn more about current ethics guidelines and applications. Speech-language-hearing professionals are faced with ethical issues that may result in ethical dilemmas. Dilemmas may include a wide variety of issues, such as autonomy, beneficence, nonmaleficence, and justice. Ethical principles, morals, values, beliefs, and law often factor into a decision-making process used by a professional. Ethical principles have remained relatively constant over time, but the codes of ethics for professional organizations/associations have been changed as new ethical issues have evolved. The changes in the codes of ethics will continually challenge the professional to remain informed about current principles and rules that can impact practice.

Conceptual Approach and Method of Instruction

The first four chapters of this book are written to provide theoretical underpinnings and a historical overview and to lay the foundation for ethical decision making. It is important for all readers to have reviewed these chapters prior to proceeding to the other chapters; it is important to use the information gleaned from those chapters while applying the case-based scenarios presented in Chapter 5 through Chapter 8. The use of case-based scenarios is helpful to describe the problem and the application of an ethical decision-making process. In this text, the codes of ethics for ASHA and AAA are used as reference points for developing case-based scenarios. The intent is for readers to utilize these case scenarios as tools for applying the steps in ethical decision making. Faculty at a university and team facilitators within a work setting are encouraged to utilize the *Instructor's Manual* to support discussions by a group through ethical decision making. In some case scenarios, more explicit questions with possible answers are provided to offer a "model," and other scenarios are presented with a basic set of questions that should lead to more problem solving by the reader.

Organization of the Text

The organization of the text includes a general orientation to professionalism and the role of ethics, followed by a discussion about the evolution of the ASHA and AAA codes of ethics. These documents are not static and will continue to evolve. The reader must not accept the use of this book as a final stop for ethics education. One must continue to monitor and remain informed about changes in the codes of ethics for professional organizations, licensing boards, state speech-language-hearing association, and employers. The codes of ethics and/or codes of conduct can overlap for each of these, but some have distinct jurisdictions over a professional.

The steps in any ethical decision-making model should be logical and applicable to a variety of situations. Important and relevant information must be gathered in a manner that is useful to others who may be called to make a decision about the ethical—or unethical—conduct of another person. These steps are illustrated in the case scenarios and further explained in the *Instructor's Manual.* A response to an ethical dilemma or scenario is not always readily available to the reader, but the case-based scenarios that are presented should prompt discussions among the readers involving logical and sound decision making.

Features

The use of case-based scenarios has been mentioned, but readers must remember that there are numerous other scenarios that could have been used. The use of "Vee" diagrams are helpful to have each case scenario analyzed and discussed in a similar manner. Being mindful of confidentiality, readers may want to develop and use scenarios that they have experienced. If other scenarios are used by the reader, a commitment should be made to apply all steps of the ethical decision-making model. In other words, identifying and gathering documentation should not be the only step completed in the process. Partial application of an ethical decision-making process of a scenario is discouraged because it could lead to inappropriate conclusions.

Instructor's Manual

The accompanying *Instructor's Manual* establishes a pedagogical framework for facilitating ethical development. It includes a variety of innovative materials to stimulate critical thinking in the area of ethics, as well as detailed applications designed to offer solutions to selected scenarios. Also included in the *Instructor's Manual* are many illustrative diagrams, sample discussion topics, and test items.

The authors of this book all share a strong interest in ethics education. All have been involved in teaching, research, and direct client care that support their expertise in writing this book. The authors shared a common goal to develop a text that will help support the education of professionals to develop effective ethical decision-making strategies. The book and instructor's manual can be used to facilitate education for students, university faculty, and clinically based and educationally based professionals.

David L. Irwin, PhD, CCC-SLP, is Professor and Head for the Department of Clinical Services and Director of the Children's Center in the School of Allied Health Professions at Louisiana State University Health Sciences Center in Shreveport. He holds adjunct appointment in the Speech-Language Pathology Program at LSUHSC-Shreveport and also teaches in the Master of Health Sciences Program. He has taught at several universities in Oklahoma and Louisiana with his primary interests being language development and language disorders, professional issues, and research methods. His clinical experiences include public schools, a state institution for juvenile delinquent males, hospitals, home health, private practice, and universities. He has served as President of the Louisiana Speech-Language-Hearing Association (LSHA), is a Fellow of the American Speech-Language-Hearing Association (ASHA), and has co-presented with Dr. Mary Pannbacker in the area of ethics.

Mary Pannbacker, PhD, CCC-SLP, is Professor in the Speech-Language Pathology Program in the Department of Rehabilitation Sciences at the School of Allied Health Professions at LSUHSC-Shreveport. Her professional experience includes teaching at universities in Pennsylvania, New York, and Texas. She is a Fellow of ASHA and is a recipient of the Service Award of the American Cleft Palate Craniofacial Association. She has served as President of the LSHA. Currently, she serves as Legislative Councilor from Louisiana to ASHA and Editor of the LSHA Newsletter. She has numerous presentations and publications related to cleft palate, voice disorders, and professional issues.

Thomas W. Powell, PhD, CCC-SLP, is Professor and Head of the Department of Rehabilitation Sciences, housed in the School of Allied Health Professions, at LSUHSC-Shreveport. His primary areas of interest include phonetics and phonology, aphasia, multilingualism, measurement, and research design. He is co-editor of *Clinical Linguistics and Phonetics*, which is the official journal of the International Clinical Phonetics and Linguistics Association.

Gay T. Vekovius, MS, CCC-AUD, has recently retired from the Department of Rehabilitation Sciences in the School of Allied Health Professions at LSUHSC-Shreveport. She served on the professional licensure board for the State of Louisiana, including a term as Chair. She was President of LSHA and served on several committees and boards for ASHA. She is a Fellow of ASHA, and her interests include high-tech hearing aids, aural rehabilitation, and professional issues.

Acknowledgments

Several speech-language pathologists and audiologists contributed case studies to this book: Sharon Sanders, CCC-AUD; Darla Rakoczy, CCC-SLP; Heather Anderson, CCC-SLP; and Sandra Hayes, CCC-SLP. Special thanks are also due to others who helped with this book in different ways: Kay Davis, T. Newel Decker, David Denton, Nancy Huffman, and Glen Waguespack. The contributions of the reference librarians at LSUHSC-Shreveport are also acknowledged: Kerri Christopher, David Duggar, Leslie Fitzgerald, and Bob Wood.

 Disclaimer

All case scenarios presented in this book are fictitious and do not depict any specific individual or situation. Any resemblance to an actual situation or person is purely coincidental. Nothing in this book should be construed as legal advice. Our interpretation of ethical codes or standards should not be viewed as reflecting the official opinion of any specific professional association.

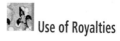 **Use of Royalties**

All royalties received by the authors from this book will be donated to the LSU Health Sciences Foundation in Shreveport to support a scholarship for a graduate student in speech-language pathology exhibiting high ethical standards and understanding of the application of these principles to clinical practice at LSUHSC-Shreveport.

Chapter 1

Professionalism and Ethics

Learning Objectives

After reading this chapter, you should be able to:

- Describe the differences between law and ethics.
- Describe the basic terms used in ethical decision making including autonomy, beneficence, nonmaleficence, and justice.
- Discuss the basic ethical principles of the ASHA and AAA codes of ethics.
- Identify the basic components of a code of conduct required by employers.
- Discuss a scenario that involves an audiologist or a speech-language pathologist experiencing an ethical dilemma.
- Identify the number of states that have a code of ethics for the professions of speech-language pathology and audiology.
- Identify the number of states that have rules and regulations for the role of support personnel.

Introduction

Ethical decision making for speech-language pathologists (SLPs) and audiologists (AUDs) is a process that involves professional issues that range from simple to complex. Professional decisions are impacted by personal morals, values, beliefs, professional judgment, client needs, and a wide variety of other factors. Given the complexity of issues and the need for balance among them, various groups or organizations have developed guidelines that govern standards of practice. These groups include but are not limited to the American Speech-Language-Hearing Association (ASHA), the American Academy of Audiology (AAA), state licensure boards, and state speech-language-hearing associations. The place of employment, too, may establish rules and regulations or codes of conduct.

It is the responsibility of each member of an organization to be knowledgeable about the current version of the code of ethics or rules governing ethical practice. Accordingly, the primary purpose of this chapter is to provide an overview of the purposes of ethics, ethical principles, and professional codes of ethics that govern clinical and research decision making.

Purposes of Ethics

According to Grodin (1995), **ethics** is "a branch of philosophy, which through formal and systematic analysis, attempts to critically examine human conduct focusing on the rightness and wrongness, goodness or harmfulness of actions" (p. 7). Horner (2003) asserts the philosophical study of morality is ethics that focuses on the normative issues and must address what "*should* be done and *why*" (p. 265). Applied ethics should include a description of the "conduct of individuals and groups, so as to prevent and resolve moral problems" (Horner, p. 265). This definition of applied ethics is apparent in the **codes of ethics** for many professional organizations (e.g., ASHA, AAA) and in the workplace because there are basic principles such as **autonomy, beneficence, nonmaleficence,** and **justice** that would guide ethical decisions.

Different subtypes of ethics can be used to guide professionals. Horner (2003) described these subgroups to include **normative ethics, metaethics, descriptive ethics, professional ethics, clinical ethics, public health ethics,** and **research ethics** (see Table 1-1). It is imperative that speech-language-hearing professionals be knowledgeable

Table 1-1 Morality and Ethics/Types of Ethics

Morality	Ethics
Widely held values of a community	Philosophical ethics studies the meaning of right/wrong, good/bad, as well as nature and justification of normative standards and moral judgments.
Broad principles or guidelines focused on human happiness, well-being, security, flourishing, and fairness	Applied ethics describes and prescribes standards of conduct for individuals and groups, so as to prevent and resolve moral problems.
Ultimate	Principle based
Universal	Other-regarding
Impartial	
Other-regarding	

Types of Ethics	
Normative ethics	What should or ought to be done
Metaethics	The nature and justification of moral judgments
Descriptive ethics	Actual values and actions
Professional ethics	Applied to particular scientific, technical, and health professions with a focus on protecting the interests of the clients served
Clinical ethics	Applied to individual clients in complex clinical situations involving uncertainty to ensure that clinicians act for the good of their clients, while respecting clients' rights to self-determination and dignity
Public health ethics	Applied to public health officials and agents who are concerned with population-based health and safety regulations (e.g., vaccinations, contagious diseases, addiction, counterbioterrorism measures)
Research ethics	Applied to those who conduct research involving human (or animal) participants to ensure the integrity of the research process and to protect the interests of participants

Note. From "Morality, Ethics, and Law: Introductory Concepts," by J. C. Horner, 2003, *Seminars in Speech and Language, 24,* 263–274. Reprinted with permission.

about how these areas are applied and impact their professions. For example, speech and hearing scientists would need to be knowledgeable about professional, clinical, and research ethics because they must respect participants' rights and ensure that they act for the good of the participants.

Horner (2003) differentiates ethics from law; professionals must understand that, although the concepts are related, they do not necessarily address all moral dilemmas in the same way. For example, Horner (2003) describes **law** as being "defined by government, based on concepts of justice and equality, minimum standard of behavior, coercive, and rules enforced by regulatory agencies and courts" (p. 270). In contrast, Horner describes ethics as "defined by an individual or community, informal guidelines for resolution, ideal or aspirational, noncoercive, and standards and exhortation by custom, professional standards, discussion and persuasion." Laws serve a purpose to create and maintain an ordered society and to protect rights, whereas ethics "refers to rules and principles (based on values) that we abide by or at least strive to abide by" (Horner, 2003, p. 272) and implies the use of reason and acting fairly for all concerned.

Ethical Principles

Ethical principles that are used to guide decision making focus primarily upon four different areas: (1) respect for autonomy, (2) beneficence, (3) nonmaleficence, and (4) justice. Horner (2003) described each of these ethical principles as identified in Table 1-2. Principles provide guidelines for action, but they do not solve problems. Professionals must review the evidence of a case and apply ethical principles to determine the appropriate course of action. Ethical principles are rarely sufficient for professionals to solve moral quandaries. Other contributing factors include use of good judgment, sound reasoning, and virtues of character (Horner, 2003).

Table 1-2 Guiding Ethical Principles

Principle	Description
Respect for autonomy (*auto*, self; *nomos*, rule)	Act so as to enhance others' self-determination; refrain from interfering with free choice; protect vulnerable persons; and foster self-determination (self-governance) as much as possible.
Beneficence (*bene*, good)	Act to benefit others; balance good results over potential harms against potential benefits.
Nonmaleficence (*mal*, bad)	Act to avoid harm; balance risks and seriousness of potential harms against potential benefits.
Justice (fairness)	Act to distribute the benefits and burdens of society fairly:
	Substantive justice: Give others what they need or deserve.
	Procedural justice: Use impartial decision-making procedures.
	Allocative justice: Distribute societal resources (such as health care) equitably.

Note. From "Morality, Ethics, and Law: Introductory Concepts," by J. C. Horner, 2003, *Seminars in Speech and Language, 24,* 263–274. Reprinted with permission.

Although the ethical principles presented by Horner (2003) are often cited, it may be beneficial to explore ethics from another perspective. The hierarchical structure of the (American Speech-Language-Hearing Association [ASHA], 2003a) Code of Ethics is examined in Figure 1-1 using the "Mind Map"® approach of Buzan and Buzan (1993).

Five primary categories were identified by qualitatively analyzing the vocabulary commonly used in the Code of Ethics utilized by ASHA (2003a). The category of human relations dominates concepts such as unfair discrimination, informed consent, unprofessional conduct, and sexual harassment. The associated principles of the ASHA Code of Ethics are given in circles. The graphic organization of these guiding ethical principles could help the professional to first determine which major area (human

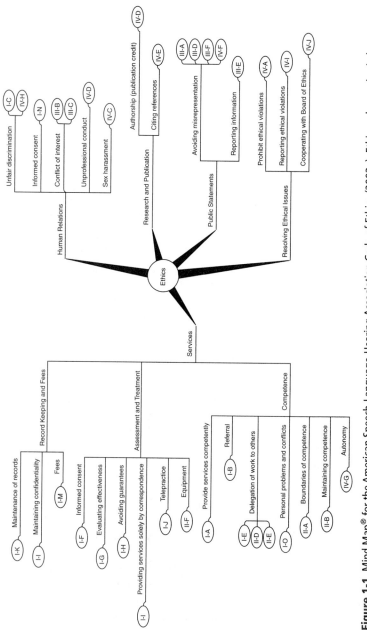

Figure 1-1 Mind Map® for the American Speech-Language-Hearing Association Code of Ethics (2003a). Ethics rules are in circles.

relations, research and publication, public statements, resolving ethical issues or service) might be considered when addressing ethical dilemmas. It is possible that an ethical dilemma could involve more than one branch and the professional would need to consult various ethical principles when making decisions. An advantage to this type of analysis is that the professional can identify and apply the relevant ethical principles of the ASHA Code of Ethics. This approach helps one to determine which areas might need documentation and evidence and in which areas faculty, students, or colleagues may need further education.

A similar "Mind Map"® was prepared for the (American Academy of Audiology [AAA], 2003) Code of Ethics, and it is included in Figure 1-2. Both the ASHA and AAA codes of ethics involve similar issues such as conflict of interest, avoiding guarantees, and reporting ethical violations.

CASE SCENARIO 1-1

An audiologist is a member of AAA and ASHA and has been in private practice for eleven years. An otolaryngologist suggests that the audiologist conduct a speech and language evaluation of a six-year-old child. The physician and the audiologist know that the child's family does not have the financial resources for a private speech-language evaluation. It is important that the child be assigned a diagnostic code for the hearing loss that was identified by the audiologist and that this code be checked on the "charge ticket." A diagnostic code for the hearing loss and for a speech-language evaluation is checked on the "charge ticket" submitted by the otolaryngologist.

Utilizing Figure 1-1 and Figure 1-2, what are the major areas/principles that the audiologist should consider when making ethical decisions?

• The audiologist should consider the areas of services, human relations, and public statements.

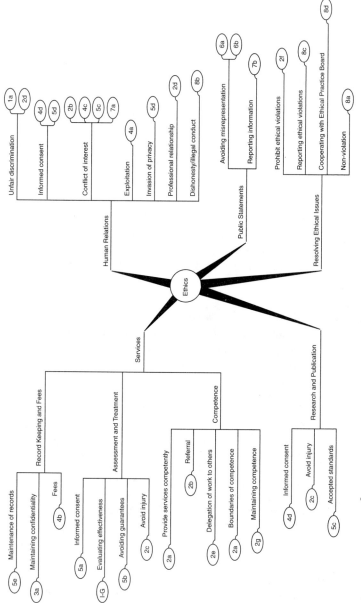

Figure 1-2 Mind Map® for the American Academy of Audiology Code of Ethics (2003). Ethics rules for the AAA are listed in the circles.

How would one justify identification of those specific areas?

- The area of services encompasses competence (and boundaries of competence) and record keeping. Human relations would include reviewing dishonesty/illegal conduct. Public statements would include avoiding misrepresentation.

Which principles are at risk for being violated?

- ASHA Principle II, Rule A (boundaries of competence); ASHA Principle I, Rule A (provide services competently); ASHA Principle III, Rule A (not misrepresent credentials); and ASHA Principle III, Rule D (not misrepresent diagnostic information)
- AAA Principle 2, Rule 2a (boundaries of competence); AAA Principle 6, Rule 6a (avoiding misrepresentation); and Principle 8, Rule 8b AAA (not engage in dishonesty).

Construct a similar scenario for an ASHA-certified speech-language pathologist who is asked to conduct a hearing evaluation. Would the areas for a speech-language pathologist be the same as for the audiologist when one utilizes Figure 1-1 and Figure 1-2?

American Speech-Language-Hearing Association Code of Ethics

For over seventy years, ASHA has had a code of ethics, which has undergone several changes (see Chapter 2). ASHA members are informed about the changes in the code of ethics through several means including *The ASHA Leader* (which is published by the organization several times per year), the ASHA Web site, ASHA supplements, and continuing education (CE) activities. The most recent revision of the Code of Ethics occurred in 2003 (ASHA, 2003a) and is available for review on-line at http://www.asha.org.

The Board of Ethics for ASHA is charged with "the responsibility to interpret, administer, and enforce the Code of Ethics for the Association" (ASHA, 2004b, p. 1). All members should review the procedures utilized by the

Board of Ethics to keep current about changes in procedures and the process necessary to file a complaint.

The Code of Ethics contains four Principles of Ethics that provide the underlying moral basis for decision making. Principle of Ethics I focuses primarily upon the welfare of persons served, both professionally and in research, as well as the humane treatment of animals. Principle of Ethics II relates to the highest level of professional competence including holding the appropriate Certificate of Clinical Competence (CCC) and the proper use and maintenance of equipment. Principle of Ethics III primarily involves promoting public understanding about the professions including the dissemination of research findings and scholarly activities. Principle of Ethics IV focuses primarily upon the relationships professionals often encounter and acceptance of the self-imposed standards (ASHA, 2004b).

American Academy of Audiology Code of Ethics

The AAA was established in 1988 and has subsequently adopted a code of ethics for its members, with the most recent revision being 2003. The AAA Code of Ethics, as stated in its preamble, "specifies professional standards that allow for the proper discharge of audiologists responsibilities to those served, and that protect the integrity of the profession" (AAA, 2003, p. 1). The AAA Code of Ethics is primarily divided into two parts, which include Principles and Rules followed by the process for enforcement of principles and rules (i.e., procedures for the management of alleged violations).

Principle 1 of the AAA Code of Ethics (2003) addresses the provision of professional services and research. Principle 2 involves the standards of professional competence for which members are qualified by education and experience. Principle 3 relates to confidentiality of information and records. Principle 4 includes the provision of services and products that are in the best interest of those served. Principle 5 relates to the accuracy of information shared during research projects, services, and products. Principle 6 includes the need to comply with AAA's use of public statements or publications. Principle 7 includes rules about the use of professional or commercial affiliations. Principle 8 includes rules relative to dignity of the profession and acceptance of the self-imposed standards.

Similar to ASHA, AAA has an Ethical Practice Board that is charged with upholding its Code of Ethics. Again, all members of the AAA should regularly review this information to be knowledgeable about the changes and possible courses of action should a complaint be filed with the Ethical Practice Board. This information is disseminated to the membership of the AAA through various publications and supplements (AAA, 2003).

State Speech-Language-Hearing Association Codes of Ethics

State speech-language-hearing associations (SSLHAs) have the option of being affiliated with ASHA. If the SSLHA affiliates with ASHA, then it is required to adopt a code of ethics. All fifty states, the District of Columbia, and the Overseas Association of Communication Sciences have an official affiliation with ASHA (ASHA, 2003b). According to Vekovius (1996), the code of ethics governing professionals at the state level is quite similar to ASHA's and a mechanism exists to keep it current by requiring SSLHAs to renew their affiliation based on cyclical rotation provided by ASHA.

SSLHAs vary in governing structure, and the process for enforcing the code of ethics for a particular state will depend on the structure. Because SSLHAs do not award certification or licensure, the most severe penalty imposed is revocation of membership; however, other types of reprimand may follow the procedures outlined by ASHA and AAA.

State Licensure Laws

All fifty states regulate the professions of speech-language pathology and/or audiology (ASHA, 2005). The District of Columbia does not regulate SLPs or AUDs, and four states (Colorado, Idaho, Michigan, and South Dakota) do not regulate SLPs. Colorado regulates audiology via registration, "which is NOT required to practice the professions. However, persons who want to use the protected titles must meet certain requirements and be registered" (ASHA, n.d.). Vekovius (1996) found that most states with licensure laws have professional standards based on ASHA's Code of Ethics. Because state licensure laws may reflect the ASHA Certificate of Clinical Competence, most of the rules and/or regulations utilized by states either adopt the wording of ASHA's Code of Ethics exactly or use it "as the basis of professional conduct" (Vekovius, 1996, p. 4). When state licensure laws adopt nationally recognized standards of professional conduct, one can move from state to state with less confusion.

The regulation of support personnel by states has recently gained more attention. According to ASHA (2004a), there are thirty-three states that officially regulate the use of support personnel. Nine of those states require licensure; the other twenty-four states regulate support personnel through registration. Four states do not have support personnel directly regulated; however, SLPs and AUDs who use support personnel are required to observe specific supervisory guidelines (ASHA, 2004a). Regardless of the type of education, experience, and amount of supervision required for support personnel, ethical issues and dilemmas are ultimately the responsibility of the supervising SLP and/or AUD.

Rules and Regulations for Place of Employment
Corporate ethics is the practice of shared values and includes a code of business conduct that holds personnel at an employment setting to basic standards and ethics. The code of business conduct applies to all employees and is used to guide ethical decision making for the employer/employees (Chindex, 2005). Like many licensing boards, failure to follow the code of business conduct can result in sanctions for the employer, employee, and/or the company.

Standards of conduct are applicable to all employees (even those under temporary contracts) because they represent the employer. Schools, hospitals, and corporations typically require that each employee sign a **code of conduct** when beginning employment. Some organizations require that employees complete an annual review of corporate ethics and sign that they agree to abide by them (Louisiana State University Health Sciences Center–Shreveport [LSUHSC-S], 2005).

Codes of business conduct may encompass many of the same principles that are part of licensure boards, state associations, and national organizations. For example, the Maxis Health System Compliance Program (Marian Hospital, 2005) requires that employees adhere to a standard of conduct that "is critical for us to appreciate the relationship with those we serve as a sacred trust which we take seriously" (p. 2). Recognizing that ethical **dilemmas** are a part of life, corporations and health care systems recognize that a written and well-defined policy of a standard of conduct will "focus on making the right choice for the right reason" (Marian Hospital, 2005, p. 2).

Failure to comply with the standard of conduct for a business can result in "censure by the employee, demotion or re-assignment of the individual involved, suspension with or without pay or benefits and termination of the individual's employment" (Chindex, 2005, p. 10). Like professional organizations and licensure boards, corporations often have a committee that deals with reviewing complaints about ethical conduct of employees and possible courses of action.

Summary

Speech-language pathologists and audiologists have the responsibility to be knowledgeable about ethical principles and rules that govern their practice. For some, this may include ASHA, state licensure laws, and state speech-language hearing associations. For others, it may involve AAA, ASHA, and a code of conduct for their place of employment. Whatever the situation for the professional, it is imperative to keep current and apply the ethical principles and rules in a manner that involves ethical decision

14 Chapter 1

making. The four primary areas of ethics include: autonomy, beneficence, nonmaleficence, and justice as described by Horner (2003). Being knowledgeable about laws that govern practice is important, but that knowledge alone would not be sufficient for effective decision making.

References

American Academy of Audiology. (2003). *Code of ethics, procedures, rules & penalties.* Retrieved at http://www.audiology.org.

American Speech-Language-Hearing Association (ASHA). (2003a). Code of ethics. *ASHA Supplement, 23,* 13–15.

American Speech-Language-Hearing Association. (2003b). *Procedures for recognition of state associations.* Retrieved at http://www.asha.org.

American Speech-Language-Hearing Association. (2004a). *Speech-language pathology assistants: Frequently asked questions.* Retrieved at http://www.asha.org.

American Speech-Language-Hearing Association. (2004b). *Statement of practices and procedures of the Board of Ethics.* Retrieved at http://www.asha.org.

American Speech-Language-Hearing Association. (n.d.). *State licensure trends.* Retrieved at http://www.asha.org/about/legislation-advocacy/state/state-license.htm.

Buzan, T., & Buzan, B. (1993). *The Mind Map® book.* New York: Plume.

Chindex. (2005). *Chindex code of business conduct.* Retrieved at http://www.chindex.com.

Grodin, M. A. (Ed.). (1995). *Meta medical ethics: The philosophical foundation of bioethics.* Boston: Kluwer Academic Publishers.

Horner, J. (2003). Morality, ethics, and law: Introductory concepts. *Seminars in Speech and Language, 24,* 263–274.

Louisiana State University Health Sciences Center–Shreveport (LSUHSC-S). (2005). *Code of conduct.* Retrieved at http://www.sh.lsuhsc.edu.

Marian Hospital. (2005). *Standard of conduct.* Retrieved at http://www.marianhospital.org.

Vekovius, G. (1996). *Professional standards of behavior in state licensure laws.* Unpublished manuscript.

Chapter 2

Evolution of the ASHA Code of Ethics

Learning Objectives

After reading this chapter, you should be able to:

- Discuss the historical background that led to the creation of the first ASHA Code of Ethics.
- Explain the reasons for changes in the ASHA Code of Ethics.
- Identify the major changes in the 2003 Code of Ethics.
- Describe the evolution of selected areas of the Code of Ethics.
- Discuss ASHA's activities related to ethics.
- Define terms used in the chapter.
- Identify future ethical issues.

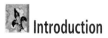 Introduction

Ethics were critical in what eventually became the professions of speech-language pathology and audiology. When ASHA was founded as the American Academy of Speech Correction in 1925, the establishment of a code of ethics was identified as a primary reason for the organization (Paden, 1970). This was related to concerns about unprofessional practices, exorbitant fees, and guarantees. To address the changes that have occurred over the years, the Code of Ethics has been revised fourteen times. A chronology of these revisions is presented in Table 2-1.

This chapter provides information about the first ASHA Code of Ethics, revisions of the Code of Ethics, the 2003

Table 2-1 Chronology of Revisions of ASHA's Code of Ethics

1930	First Code of Ethics
	Prohibited treatment entirely by correspondence
	Listed nine unethical practices
1952	Modified unethical practices from nine to ten; addressed confidentiality and supervision
	Referral and suggestion of financial conflict of interest
	Included reasonable statement of prognosis
	Organized into three divisions based on ethical responsibilities
1965	Revised preamble
1971	Addressed discrimination
1975	Considered conflict of interest
1977	Changed from avoiding advertisements to providing public statements and announcements
1979	Adopted gender equality (nonsexist language usage), product dispensing, informed consent
	Authorship
	Continuing professional development
	Divided into three categories: principles of ethics, ethical prescriptions, and matters of professional propriety
1986	Added Ethical Prescriptions to Principle of Ethics VI (standards and responsibilities to the profession)
1990	Reduced Principles of Ethics from six to five
1991	Essentially unchanged from 1990

continued

Table 2-1 (Continued)

1992	Eliminated Ethical Proscriptions
	Advanced independent professional judgment, autonomy
	Eliminated Matters of Professional Propriety
	Changed fundamentals to Principles of Ethics and Rules of Ethics
	Defined misrepresentation
	Reduced Principles of Ethics from five to four
	Considered substance abuse
1993	Added Principle of Ethics IV, Rule of Ethics H expanded discrimination
1994	Reorganization of Principles of Ethics IV, Rules of Ethics A–H
2001	Modified to include:
	Avoid biased referral
	Appropriate referencing in oral and written presentations
	Sexual harassment
	Sexual misconduct with clients, students, colleagues
	Assistants
	Telecommunication/telepractice
	Personal financial interest
2003	Expanded research and scholarly activities
	Informed consent
	Confidentiality
	Humane treatment of animals
	Appropriate maintenance of research data

Code of Ethics, the evolution of selected areas, and ASHA's related ethical activities. All ASHA codes of ethics subsequent to the original 1930 Code of Ethics have been separate documents from the association's constitution and bylaws. Revisions were adopted in 1952, 1965, 1971, 1975, 1977, 1979, 1986, 1990, 1991, 1992, 1993, 1994, 2001, and 2003. The Code was revised only twice in the first thirty-five years (1948, 1965) of the association. Since then, the Code has been revised eleven times and as often as every two years (1975, 1977, 2001). Between 1990 and 1994, the Code was revised five times. Revisions of the Code brought changes in content that varied in degree. Some of these changes are summarized later in this chapter and in Table 2-1. The 1992 Code of Ethics had many changes including principles and rules related to professional autonomy, substance abuse, and scope of competence. ASHA's 2001 Code of Ethics also had several changes related to assistants, telecommunication, financial conflict of interest, plagiarism, and sexual misconduct. This most recent revision (American Speech-Language-Hearing Association [ASHA], 2003) focused on research and scholarly activities.

The First ASHA Code of Ethics

The first Code of Ethics was a section of the ASHA constitution organized by the committee on Charter Membership to exclude ". . . unscientific and unscrupulous workers. . . ." It had three sections: (1) duties of the society, (2) secrecy, and (3) unethical practices. Section 2 pertained to confidentiality of information about clients: "The obligation of secrecy so far as revelation of confidences of speech patients is concerned shall be regarded as a duty of members" (as cited in Paden, 1970, p. 74; Silverman, 1983, p. 220). There were nine unethical practices, which are listed in Table 2-2. These are activities that should not be done because they are wrong.

Table 2-2 Unethical Practices Listed in the 1930 ASHA Code of Ethics

1. To guarantee to cure any disorder of speech.
2. To offer in advance to refund any part of a person's tuition if his disorder of speech is not arrested.
3. To make "rash promises," difficult of fulfillment, in order to secure pupils or patients.
4. To extend the time of treatment beyond the time when one should recognize his inability to effect further improvement.
5. To employ blatant or untrustworthy methods of self-advertising.
6. To advertise to correct disorders entirely by correspondence.
7. To seek self-advancement by attacking the work of other members of the Society in such a way as might injure their standing and reputation. Reproach or criticism should be sympathetically discussed with the member involved.
8. For persons who do not hold a medical degree to attempt to deal exclusively with speech patients requiring medical treatment without the advice or the authority of a physician.
9. To charge exorbitant fees for treatment.

Note. From *A History of the American Speech and Hearing Association,* by E. P. Paden, 1970, Washington, DC: American Speech and Hearing Association; *Legal Aspects of Speech-Language Pathology and Audiology,* by F. H. Silverman, 1983, Englewood Cliffs, NJ: Prentice Hall.

Revisions

The Code of Ethics is not static and has been revised as needed in response to professional practice, trends in code violations, and suggestions from ASHA members and staff. The first Code of Ethics remained virtually unchanged for eighteen years until 1948. At that time, the Committee on Ethical Practice became one of the major standing committees of the association. The committee was responsible for preparing revisions of the Code of Ethics and for investigating charges of alleged ethical misconduct (Paden, 1970). The Code of Ethics did not become a document separate from the constitution until 1952. The 1952 revision of the Code of Ethics (American Speech and Hearing Association [ASHA], 1952) described the ethical responsibilities of members relative to client relations. These responsibilities included welfare of clients and appropriate qualifications for clinicians, responsibilities to other professionals, and obligations to society. Unethical practices were expanded into a list of ten unethical practices. Additions to the previous unethical practices were related to supervision, confidentiality, and financial conflict of interest. Duties of the Committee on Ethical Practice were to review alleged ethical violations. An introduction was added to the 1952 Code of Ethics that described ethical responsibilities of members and classified these responsibilities. "The American Speech and Hearing Association is composed of persons having varying interests and professional duties, but certain broad ethical principles apply to the entire membership. The application of these principles to individual cases will depend on the particular circumstances of the professional duties and status of the persons involved" (p. 255). The ethical responsibilities were related to ASHA members, other professionals, and the public. After 1952, none of the revised codes included a list of unethical practices, that is, what actions may not be done because they are wrong. This information is implied in the rules, which state when actions are right.

From 1979 to 1991, the Code of Ethics had three fundamental rules of ethical conduct: Principles of Ethics,

Table 2-3 Description of Fundamental Rules of Ethical Conduct (ASHA, 1979)

Principles of Ethics—Six principles serve as a basis for the ethical evaluation of professional conduct and form the underlying basis for the Code of Ethics. Individuals subscribing to this Code shall observe these principles as affirmative obligations under all conditions of professional activities.

Ethical Proscriptions—Ethical proscriptions are formal statements of prohibitions that are derived for the Principles of Ethics.

Matters of Professional Propriety—Matters of professional propriety represent guidelines of conduct designed to promote the public interest and thereby better inform the public and particularly the person in need of speech-language pathology and audiology services to the availability and the rules regarding the delivery of these services.

Ethical Proscriptions, and Matters of Professional Propriety. These categories are described in Table 2-3. Principles serve as the foundations for rules and are more general in nature. Rules are more specific and indicate certain actions that should be done because they are right (Strand, Yorkston, & Miller, 1998). Since 1992 (ASHA), the fundamentals of ethical conduct have been described by Principles of Ethics and by Rules of Ethics. "Rules of Ethics are specific statements of minimally acceptable conduct or of prohibitions and are applicable to all individuals" (p. 1).

The 2001 Code of Ethics (ASHA, 2001a) had several additions and/or modifications. These changes were related to representation of credentials of assistants, delegation of tasks to assistants, provision of clinical services by correspondence and telecommunication, referrals based on personal financial interest, sexual harassment, sexual activities with persons over whom one exercises professional authority, and plagiarism (Huffman, 2002).

2003 Ethics Code

The major changes in the 2003 Code of Ethics were related to research and scholarly activities (Mustain, 2003). The Preamble (ASHA, 2003) was modified to include "speech, language, and hearing scientists" and expanded the fundamentals of ethical conduct to include "research and scholarly activities" (p. 1). Appendix A provides an operational classification of the 2003 Code of Ethics. The

Preamble sets the general context for the Code of Ethics. Its primary goal is "... the preservation of the highest standards of integrity and ethical principles ... " (p. 13). The Preamble describes the fundamental principles and rules. It contains no enforceable rules but indicates that "... any violation of the spirit and purpose of this Code shall be considered unethical" (p. 13).

The Principles of Ethics form the underlying basis for the Code of Ethics: welfare of persons served professionally, competence, public statements and announcements, and professionalism. These principles are affirmative obligations and should be observed during all professional activities. Within each Principle of Ethics, there are Rules of Ethics, which are specific statements of minimally acceptable professional conduct or prohibitions that are applicable to all individuals.

The Rules of Ethics are specific and constitute a list of standards for all speech-language pathologists (SLPs) and audiologists (AUDs). The Rules inform SLPs and AUDs of their responsibilities to refer, provide, inform, or document and, on the other hand, to avoid negative actions such as misrepresentation, discrimination, or sexual misconduct.

All SLPs and AUDs should thoroughly study the Code of Ethics to be familiar with current ethical standards and to avoid unethical practices and ensure ethical conduct. Every individual who is an ASHA member, nonmembers with the Certificate of Clinical Competence, applicants for membership or certification, and students seeking to fulfill certification standards must abide by the principles and rules of the Code of Ethics. These principles and rules address issues that are encountered by SLPs and AUDs in a variety of settings and address problems that have broad application such as incompetence, sexual misconduct, substance abuse, conflicts of interest, treatment guarantees, and plagiarism, to name a few. These issues are discussed in the next section, "Evolution of Selected Areas." Speech-language pathologists and audiologists should devote extra attention to those parts of the Code of Ethics that address their particular area of work. For example, individuals involved in research should be especially knowledgeable about the principles and rules related to research and scholarly activities in addition to the rest of the Code of Ethics. These principles and rules are listed in Table 2-4.

Table 2-4 ASHA Code of Ethics: References to Research (ASHA, 2003)

Individuals shall honor their responsibility to hold paramount the welfare of persons they serve professionally or participants in *research* and scholarly activities and shall treat animals involved in *research* in a humane manner (Principle of Ethics I).

Individuals shall not discriminate in the delivery of professional services or the conduct of *research* and scholarly activities on the basis of race or ethnicity, gender, age, religion, national origin, sexual orientation, or disability (Principle of Ethics I, Rule C).

Individuals shall fully inform the persons they serve of the nature and possible effects of services rendered and products dispensed, and they shall inform participants in *research* about the possible effects of their participation in *research* conducted (Principle of Ethics I, Rule F).

Individuals shall adequately maintain and appropriately secure records of professional services rendered, *research*, and scholarly activities conducted, and products dispensed and shall allow access to these records only when authorized or when required by law (Principle of Ethics I, Rule K).

Individuals shall not reveal, without authorization, any professional or personal information about identified persons served professionally or identified participants involved in *research* and scholarly activities unless required by law to do so, or unless doing so is necessary to protect the welfare of the person or the community or otherwise required by law (Principle of Ethics I, Rule L).

Individuals shall not charge for services not rendered, nor shall they misrepresent services rendered, products dispensed, or *research* and scholarly activities conducted (Principle of Ethics I, Rule M).

Individuals shall use persons in *research* or as subjects of teaching demonstrations only with their informed consent (Principle of Ethics I, Rule N).

Individuals shall not require or permit their professional staff to provide services or conduct *research* activities that exceed the staff member's competence, level of education, training, and experience (Principle of Ethics II, Rule E).

Individuals shall ensure that all equipment used in the provision of services or to conduct *research* and scholarly activities is in proper working order and is properly calibrated (Principle of Ethics II, Rule F).

Individuals shall honor their responsibility to the public by promoting public understanding of the professions, by supporting the development of services designed to fulfill the unmet needs of the public, and by providing accurate information in all communications involving any aspect of the professions, including dissemination of *research* findings and scholarly activities (Principle of Ethics III).

continued

Table 2-4 (Continued)

Individuals shall not misrepresent their credentials, competence, education, training, experience, or scholarly *research* contributions (Principle of Ethics III, Rule A).

Individuals shall not misrepresent diagnostic information, *research*, services rendered, or products dispensed; neither shall they engage in any scheme to defraud in connection with obtaining payment or reimbursement for such services or products (Principle of Ethics III, Rule D).

Individuals' statements to the public shall provide accurate information about the nature and management of communication disorders about the professions, about professional services, and about *research* and scholarly activities (Principle of Ethics III, Rule E).

Individuals' statements to the public—advertising, announcing, and marketing their professional services, reporting *research* results, and promoting products—shall adhere to prevailing professional standards and shall not contain misrepresentations (Principle of Ethics III, Rule F).

Individuals shall assign credit only to those who have contributed to a publication, presentation, or product. Credit shall be assigned in proportion to the contribution and only with the contributor's consent (Principle of Ethics IV, Rule D).

Individuals shall reference the source when using other person's ideas, *research* results, or products in written, oral, or any other media presentation or summary (Principle of Ethics IV, Rule E).

Individuals' statements to colleagues about professional services, *research* results, and products shall adhere to prevailing professional standards and shall contain no misrepresentations (Principle of Ethics IV, Rule F).

Evolution of Selected Areas

The various revisions of the Code of Ethics can be reviewed relative to changes motivated by factors related to the evolution of society and the professions of speech-language pathology and audiology. Several areas have had important changes in content over the years. Among these are telepractice, conflict of interest, product dispensing, sexual misconduct, misrepresentation, substance abuse, scope of competence, research and related scholarly activities, teaching, and discrimination.

Telepractice

Telepractice is the application of telecommunication technology to deliver professional services at a distance by linking client to clinician, or clinician to clinician, for assessment, intervention and/or consultation (ASHA, 2001a). It has the advantages of "(1) reducing barriers to access and/or specialized expertise; (2) being cost effective;

(3) enhancing provider productivity and/or effectiveness; and (4) creating additional value/benefits for the health care provider and/or the consumer (e.g., reduced travel time and costs)." In addition, outcomes may be enhanced through telepractice (ASHA, 2005c). In 2001, ASHA added a Rule of Ethics related to telepractice, which states, "Individuals may practice by telecommunication (for example, telehealth/e-health), where not prohibited by law" (ASHA, 2001a, p. 2). Telepractice challenged the traditional view of clinical service as involving face-to-face encounters between clinicians and clients. There are other ethical issues related to telepractice such as privacy and confidentiality, technical competence, standard of care, privacy, informed consent, and the use of support personnel (Denton, 2003; Denton & Gladstone, 2005).

Conflict of Interest

A guiding principle for SLPs and AUDs is that they shall avoid conflicts of interest. **Conflict of interest** is a term that includes a wide range of behaviors and circumstances involving personal gain or financial interest (Bradley, 1995). The ASHA (2004b) Board of Ethics defined conflicts of interest as "situations where personal and/or financial considerations compromise judgment in any professional activity (e.g., clinical service, research, consultation, instruction, administration) or where the situation may appear to provide the potential for professional judgment to be compromised" (p. 47). A conflict of interest occurs when an SLP or an AUD loses objectivity, thus compromising professional decisions. Some conflicts of interest are obvious; others may be subtle. Potential conflicts of interest include self-dealing or utilizing commercial enterprises in which one has a financial interest, and self-referral or referring clients between two work settings, both of which employ the same clinician. A conflict of interest could also occur when a clinician draws clients for private practice from his or her primary place of employment (ASHA, 2001b). Other examples of conflicts of interest include but are not limited to industry financial support of graduate students, financing development of professional products, sponsorship of presentations at professional meetings, continuing education outside professional meetings, business development funds, and partnership points (Jacobson, 2002). The term conflict of interest first appeared in the 1975 Code of Ethics, which included a specific rule that "...the ASHA member ... must guard against conflicts of professional interest." The 2003 Code (III, C) prohibits individuals from referral on the basis of any personal financial interest. In addition, the Board of Ethics provided an Issues in Ethics Statement about conflicts of professional interest (ASHA, 1993) and revised statements in 2002 and 2004. The Board of Ethics (ASHA, 2004b) advises that "Individuals must remain aware of the potential for conflicts of professional interest and take initiative to manage, disclose, or resolve potential conflict of interest situations appropriately" (p. 48).

ASHA journals require authors to disclose any real or potential conflicts of interest that could be perceived as having an influence. Potential conflicts of interest, also known as *dual commitments*, include financial interests in a test or procedure, and funding by an equipment or materials manufacturer for product-oriented outcomes research. There are also other actual or potential conflicts associated with research. These conflicts are related to authorship problems such as repetitive publication, honorary or ghost authorship, and order of authorship. Self-referral is another aspect of conflict of interest. Drawing cases for private practice from one's primary place of employment has been recognized by the Board of Ethics as a potential conflict of interest (ASHA, 2001b). Speech-language pathologists and audiologists should ". . . not involve themselves in activities that conflict with the best interests of the professions or the best interest of the persons served" (pp. 69–70).

Product Dispensing

The direct sale of products, including hearing aids, by ASHA members was prohibited by the association until a legal decision in 1978 that prohibited professional organizations from denying their members the right to provide services or products to the public (*National Society of Professional Engineers v. State of New York,* 1978). Since that time, SLPs and AUDs have increased their role in dispensing products such as augmentative communication devices and hearing aids. The 1979, 1985, and 1986 codes of ethics contained specific standards related to dispensing products. For example, products must be part of a comprehensive rehabilitation program; fees for services must be independent of the product; clients should be free to choose the source of services and products; price information must be made available; and the effectiveness of product must be determined. Subsequent codes place product dispensing in a broader context. Dispensing of products has the potential for conflicts of interest, which are prohibited by the ASHA Code of Ethics, Principle III, Rule B (2003). There are several actual or potential conflicts of interest related to product dispensing by SLPs and AUDs. These areas include commercial interest in a product company; social relationships with commercial enterprises; and rebates, gifts, and awards for dispensing products (Hawkins, 2000). There are also conflicts of interest in product-oriented research related to documenting the efficacy of products. The employment of SLPs and AUDs by manufacturers of products to conduct and report outcomes of research also creates an actual or potential conflict of interest.

Ethical issues relative to dispensing hearing aids have been considered by Hawkins (2000), Jacobson (2002), Kirkwood (2003), Liang (2000), and Metz (2000). The role of SLPs as manufacturers' representatives for augmentative communication devices has also been considered (Woltosz, Bristow, Fromkin, & Romich, 1994). ASHA (n.d.) also addresses presentation and publication of product-oriented research. This policy indicates that ASHA is a noncommercial forum unless specifically designated. It also states: "Individuals should refrain from the use of brand names and specific product endorsements whenever possible. Under no circumstances should the Association's podium be used as a place for direct promotion of a speaker's product, services, or monetary self-interest."

Sexual Misconduct

There was no reference in the Code of Ethics to sexual misconduct or sexual harassment until 2001 (ASHA, 2001a). In the 2001 and subsequent codes, there are two specific references related to sexual misconduct. Principle of Ethics IV, Rules B and C, state: "Individuals shall not engage in dishonesty, fraud, deceit, misrepresentation, sexual harassment, or any other form of conduct that adversely reflects on the professional's or on the individual's fitness to serve persons professionally. Individuals shall not engage in sexual activities with clients or students over whom they exercise professional authority." Sexual harassment is sexual solicitation, physical advances, or verbal or nonverbal conduct that is sexual in nature (Canter, Bennett, Jones, & Nagy, 1999). It includes practices ranging from direct requests for sexual favors to workplace conditions that create a hostile environment for persons of either gender, including same-sex harassment (Civil Rights Act of 1964). The law generally protects individuals from sexual harassment in the workplace. Sexual harassment applies only to conduct that occurs in connection with professional activities such as teaching, research, and providing continuing education seminars or workshops and in daily professional interactions with others, including clients and colleagues.

Misrepresentation

Misrepresentation is any untrue statement(s) that is (are) likely to mislead. It also includes failure to provide any information that should be considered (ASHA, 1992). In other words, *misrepresentation* refers to reporting only an arbitrary or biased selection of information, which is sometimes referred to as *trimming* (Ingham, 2003). The term *misrepresentation* first appeared in the 1979 Code of Ethics and was related to misrepresentation of credentials: ". . . Individuals must not misrepresent their training or competence" (ASHA, 1979, p. 26). In addition, there was a provision that ". . . statements providing information about professional services and products must not contain representations or claims that are false, deceptive, or misleading." Subsequent codes (ASHA, 1986, 1991) included these provisions. In 1992, the rule about professional services and products was changed to ". . . Individuals shall not misrepresent diagnostic information, services rendered, or products dispensed or engage in any scheme or activity to defraud in connection with obtaining payment or reimbursement for such services or products."

Substance Abuse

There was no reference in the Code of Ethics to substance abuse until the 1992 Code. This Rule of Ethics indicated that members should withdraw from professional practice when substance abuse or an emotional or mental disability adversely affects the quality of services they render. This rule has been continued but was modified in 1994 to include obtaining treatment for these problems and, where appropriate, withdrawing from the affected areas of practice (ASHA, 1994).

Scope of Competence

Being a competent SLP or AUD means having the education and qualifications to perform a variety of tasks within the **scope of practice** for each of the professions, as well as understanding when it is appropriate to provide services or to refer a client (ASHA, 2001c, 2004d; Canter et al., 1999). The latter are addressed in ASHA's (2003) Code of Ethics, Principle of Ethics I, Rule B, which states that "individuals shall use every resource including referral when appropriate . . .," while Principle of Ethics II, Rule G, indicates that "services or products will be provided . . . only when benefit can reasonably be expected." This may be more related to client factors (prognosis) than competence per se. It has been suggested by Epstein and Hundert (2002) that a more comprehensive, evidence-based assessment of professional competence may improve professional practice and education because some important areas of practice are underemphasized. These areas include interpersonal skills, lifelong learning, professionalism, and integration of knowledge into clinical practice. Several strategies were suggested for assessment of professional competence. Among these strategies were clinical reasoning in situations involving clinical uncertainty, exercises to assess use of the professional literature, teamwork exercises, assessments by clients, peer assessment of professionalism, portfolios, videotapes, and mentored self-assessment. The term *scope of competence* first appeared in the 1992 Code of Ethics, which specified that individuals may only practice in areas in which they are competent based on their education, training, and experience. This Rule of Ethics restricts practice to one's area of competence.

Research and Related Scholarly Activities

Ethical standards for research have changed over time. **Informed consent** for protection of human subjects and vulnerable populations did not exist until the last half of the twentieth century. For example, twenty-two normally fluent children who were orphans at the Soldiers and Sailors Orphan's Home in Davenport, Iowa, were taught to stutter (Annett, 2002; Dyer, 2001). Ambrose and Yairi (2002) believe that the study "... should be viewed within the common standards of the period that there was no evidence of intent to harm, and that the objective of increasing disfluent speech should not be confused with instilling chronic stuttering in normally fluent children" (p. 201). It is obvious that such a study would not be permitted under current ethical standards.

Ethical conduct of research is fundamental to research activities and ultimately to the advancement of knowledge (Ingham, 2003). Research requires knowledge about scientific methods and the responsible conduct of research. The proliferation of research in speech-language pathology and audiology has increased interest in ethics related to research. Changes in technology have expanded issues such as product-oriented research, plagiarism, and copyright infringement (ASHA, 2002; Sininger, Marsh, Walden, & Wilber, 2003).

Changes in the Code of Ethics relative to research are apparent in the content of various revisions. Relevant provisions include disseminating the results of research and promoting research in the 1952 Code of Ethics (ASHA, 1952). The 1979 Code (ASHA, 1979) and subsequent codes include statements about informed consent and authorship: "Individuals shall fully inform subjects participating in research or teaching activities of the nature and possible effects of those activities" (p. 25), and "Individuals should assign credit to those who have contributed to a publication in proportion to their contribution" (p. 26). Informed consent means that a research participant makes an autonomous, voluntary decision about participation in the absence of coercion or undue influence (Ingham, 2003). Authorship should accurately reflect the contribution of the individual(s) to the work (American Psychological Association [APA], 2001). Furthermore, ethical responsibilities should be interpreted to include the ethical treatment of all collaborators, assistants, students, and employees associated with research activities (McCartney, 2002).

The 2001 Code (ASHA, 2001a) included a provision about reference citations: "Individuals shall reference the source when using other persons' ideas, research, presentation, or products in written, oral, or any other media presentation or summary" (p. 67). Failure to cite the work of another correctly could lead to a breach of the Code of Ethics and even legal action (ASHA, 2002). The appearance of plagiarism can be precluded by correct citation of references. This includes workshop presentations as well as handouts and slides used in professional presentations. ASHA's referencing standards are based on recommendations and guidelines of the *Publication Manual of the American Psychological Association* (APA, 2001).

The 2003 Code of Ethics (ASHA) was modified to expand sections related to research and scholarship that were not specifically addressed in earlier codes (Mustain, 2003). The revised standards contained expanded sections related to authorship, protection of humans or animals in research, provisions about copyrighted materials, oral commitment, and conflicts of interest (Peach, 2003). The seventeen specific statements dealing with research are listed in Table 2-4. Ingham (2003) states that ASHA's standards of research ethics are "woefully short of providing the kinds of guiding principles needed to help researchers and research students navigate the RCR (responsible conduct of research) labyrinth, avoiding the twists and turns of research misconduct" (p. 332). More recently, Ingham and Horner (2004) stated that "ASHA's Code of Ethics provides a modicum of guidance related to research ethics" (p. 24). ASHA's Issues in Ethics Statement "Ethics in Research and Professional Practice" (ASHA, 2002) provides examples of ethical issues related to research including the rights and welfare of participants in research, responsibilities of researchers, honesty in conducting and reporting research, and plagiarism. Issues important in conducting research with human subjects include informed consent, confidentiality, and privacy of data and client records, risks and benefits, institutional review boards, adherence to study protocol, and proper conduct of the study (Ingham, 2003). Researchers have several ethical responsibilities: ethical treatment of all collaborators, assistants, students, and employees; appropriate authorship; and acknowledgment of sources in all presentations, reports, and publications (ASHA, 2002).

Teaching

The ethical responsibility of teaching is addressed indirectly in Principle of Ethics I of the Code of Ethics (ASHA, 2003), which states: "Individuals shall honor their responsibility to hold paramount the welfare of persons they serve professionally . . . " (p. 1). Other standards related to these ethical responsibilities include confidentiality, supervision, delegation of activities, referral, competence, and continuing education. Consideration should be given to (1) understanding concepts such as justice, dignity, privacy, virtue, right and good, ethical principles, and moral values; (2) the meaning of freedom to make moral choices, and the connection between thinking about ethics and personal conduct; (3) ethical reasoning about choices can be helpful, although ethical certainty is often impossible; and (4) seeking exact points of difference and attempting to solve dilemmas as much as possible by resisting false distinctions and evasions (ASHA, 2002).

Furthermore, client welfare is affected by ethical issues in education of SLPs and AUDs. Several comprehensive reviews are available on the ethics of teaching (Hamilton, 2002; Keith-Spiegel et al., 2002; Strike & Soltis, 1992; Whicker & Kronenfeld, 1994). These reviews discuss issues such as academic dishonesty, assessment of students, biased treatment of students, confidentiality, dual role relations, harassment, reference letters for students, and supervision and collaboration.

There are no specific ethical guidelines for supervisors in the ASHA (2003) Code of Ethics, but three of the Principles of Ethics are related to supervision. These are Principles I, II, and IV (McCrea & Brasseur, 2003). Moreover, supervisors play a significant and vital role in modeling ethical practice for future SLPs and AUDs (King, 2003). This includes topics such as amount of supervision, confidentiality, prerequisite competencies, evaluation of client outcomes, self-assessment, and appropriate identification to clients and students. McAllister and Lincoln (2004) believe that students and supervisors can work to support the development of each other's ethical reasoning by taking opportunities to act as critical components of ethical decision making and by taking time to work through ethical dilemmas occurring in daily clinical practices. New supervisory models have raised issues related to video supervision and the responsibility of supervisors if they are not employed by the educational facility.

Discrimination

Title VII of the Civil Rights Act of 1964 protects against **discrimination** on the basis of race, religion, or sex. There was no reference to discrimination in the ASHA Code of Ethics until 1971: "... He must not discriminate on the basis of race, religion, or sex in his professional relationships with his colleagues or clients" (p. 302). In 1979, *he* and *his* were changed to *individual* when ASHA adopted a policy requiring nonsexist language usage. National origin discrimination was prohibited under Title VI of the Civil Rights Act of 1964. Individuals are entitled to the same opportunities regardless of nationality. Title I of the Americans with Disabilities Act of 1990 prohibits discriminating against individuals with disabilities, that is, having or having had a physical or mental impairment that substantially limits and/or limits major life activities. "National origin" and "handicapping condition" were added to the Code in 1993 as a second standard related to discrimination: "Individuals shall not discriminate in their relationships with colleagues, students, and members of allied professions on the basis of race, sex, age, religion, national origin, sexual orientation, or handicapping condition" (p. 2).

An important related consideration is cultural competence, which is a perspective on service delivery so that SLPs and AUDs provide ethically appropriate services to all populations, while recognizing their own cultural/linguistic background or life experience and that of their clients and students (ASHA, 2005a). In addition, cultural competence involves activities related to hiring, teaching, evaluation, and supervision. Speech-language pathologists and audiologists must be respectful of and responsive to cultural diversity (Moxley, Mahendra, & Vega-Barachowitz, 2004). Cultural diversity results from many factors and influences including ethnicity, religious beliefs, sexual orientation, socioeconomic levels, regionalisms, age-based peer groups, educational background, and mental/physical disability (ASHA, 2004c).

Cultural and communication barriers that may negatively influence diagnosis and treatments must be overcome. The ASHA Code of Ethics (2003) is relevant to many of the issues related to cultural competency. There is guidance related to welfare of the client, discrimination, referral, scope of competence, and lifelong learning to develop the knowledge and skills required to provide culturally and linguistically appropriate services (ASHA, 2004c).

Future Issues

It is difficult to speculate about what ethical issues can be anticipated in the future. However, it is certain that ethical issues will change. As the professions of speech-language pathology and audiology continue to grow and expand, additional ethical concerns will emerge. Furthermore, ethical issues will arise in the future that are not thought of today. These issues may create gaps in existing ethical guidelines and require additional policies and guidelines. Among these issues are technology, initiating and discontinuing treatment, dysphagia, ethics consultations, and complementary and alternative treatments.

Technology

Telepractice offers the potential to extend clinical services to remote, rural, and underserved populations and to culturally and linguistically diverse populations, but it also presents numerous ethical challenges. These issues are listed in Table 2-5. Technology has also created other

Table 2-5 Ethical Issues in Telepractice

- Licensure
- Laws and regulations of jurisdictions governing professional licensing
- Technical competency
- Education and training in telepractice
- Informed consent
  - Informing clients about differences between telepractice and services delivered face-to-face
- Disclosure of potential risks and benefits
- Clinical standards
- Evaluating effectiveness of services
- Risk management: Creating a safe environment
- Privacy and confidentiality: Using transmission and documentation methods that protect privacy and ensure confidentiality
- Transmission and storage of electronic health information consistent with federal and state regulations

Note. From "Speech Language Pathologists Providing Clinical Services via Telepractice: Technical Report," by American Speech-Language-Hearing Association, 2005c, *ASHA Supplement, 25;* "Ethical and Legal Issues Related to Telepractice," by D. R. Denton, 2003, *Seminars in Speech and Language, 24*(4), pp. 313–322.

ethical dilemmas related to plagiarism, cybercheating, and the use of e-mail for clinical services and supervision (ASHA, 2002; Meline & Mata-Pistokache, 2003). Furthermore, e-mail cannot supplement direct observation of speech-language pathology and audiology practicums.

Treatment Admission and Discharge

Admission and discharge from treatment should be consistent with the ASHA Code of Ethics (2003) and guidelines for admission/discharge criteria (ASHA, 2004a). However, ethical concerns may arise about providing treatment more frequently than is appropriate and discontinuing treatments (Rao & Martin, 2004; Ulrich, 2004). The former would be overtreatment or excessive treatment. The latter may be related to the SLP or AUD believing discharge is appropriate but the client or family disagreeing; the client or family terminating treatment when the SLP or AUD believes that additional treatment would be beneficial; and/or organizational policy or funding limitations affecting treatment decisions.

Dysphagia

Several ethical issues relative to providing services for dysphagia have attracted the attention of SLPs. One issue is in regard to conducting safe and/or ethical videofluoroscopic swallowing studies (ASHA, 2004e). Two related issues requiring consideration are (1) presence of a radiologist, and (2) management and documentation.

The issue of starting or discontinuing tube feedings can be controversial especially if the client is incompetent and his or her preferences are not known (Sharp & Bryant, 2003). Disagreements about assessment and/or treatment may arise among health care providers, clients, and their families. These decisions can have profound consequences because of life and death issues (ASHA, 2005b; Blackmer, 2001).

Ethics Consultations

Ethics consultations are being used increasingly to resolve ethical problems, but little information has been reported

in the speech-language pathology and audiology literature. An ethics consultation is a service provided by an
individual consultant, team, or committee to address specific ethical issues. Its purpose is to identify, analyze, and
resolve ethical dilemmas. Ethics consultations must ensure informed consent and confidentiality (Lo, 2003;
Schneiderman et al., 2003).

Complementary and Alternative Treatment

The use of complementary and alternative treatment for
speech-language-hearing providers has grown in recent
years. It encompasses a wide range of treatments that are
outside conventional practices and generally lack sufficient evidence (Ernst, Cohen, & Stone, 2004; Helm-
Estabrooks, 2004; Lundgren, 2004). Minimal attention has
been devoted to ethical requirements for assessing the
efficacy of these treatments.

ASHA's Related Ethics Activities

ASHA's Ethical Issues Unit provides guidance, information, and advice to individuals, the association, and university programs (http://www.asha.org.about/ethics). It also
tracks trends of recurring and emerging ethical issues.
From time to time, the Board of Ethics (ASHA, 2001d) provides Issues in Ethics Statements about specific issues of
ethical conduct that are intended to increase sensitivity
and awareness. These statements are illustrative of the
Code of Ethics and may assist ethical decision making.
These issues are listed in Table 2-6.

ASHA developed the Ethics Roundtable to facilitate dis-
semination of ethical issues and to encourage discussion
among members about these issues. Originally, the Ethics
Roundtable was a column in *ASHA* but now is on ASHA's
Web site (http://www.asha.org/about/ethics). Topics from the
Ethics Roundtable are listed in Table 2-7.

In addition, ASHA's journals have policies about disclosure of conflicts of interest that require authors to
acknowledge any dual commitment. Disclosure includes

Table 2-6 Issues in Ethics Statements

ASHA Policy Regarding Support Personnel (1994)

Clinical Fellowship Supervisor's Responsibilities (2004)

Clinical Practice by Certificate Holders in the Profession in Which They Are Not Certified (2004)

Competition (2004)

Confidentiality (2004)

Conflicts of Professional Interest (2004)

Cultural Competence (2005)

Drawing Cases for Private Practice from Primary Place of Employment (2001)

Ethical Practice Inquiries: ASHA Jurisdictions (2002)

Ethics in Research and Professional Practice (2001)

Fees for Clinical Service Provided by Students (2004)

Prescription (2002)

Public Announcements and Public Statements (2002)

Representation of Service for Insurance Reimbursement or Funding (2004)

Supervision of Student Clinicians (2004)

Use of Graduate Degrees by Members and Certificate Holders (2002)

Note. From *Speech-Language-Hearing Association Issues in Ethics Statements.* Retrieved May 12, 2006, from http://www.asha.org/about/ethics/ethics_issues_index.htm.

Table 2-7 Topics from ASHA's Ethics Roundtable

Are Sales Quotes Appropriate in Clinical Settings? (1999)

Ethical Issues in Randomized Clinical Trials (1999)

Interpreting a Living Will after Stroke (1999)

Recommending an Employee with a Mixed Performance Record (2000)

The Role of Rehabilitation Services at the End of Life (1998)

To Sign or Not? Advising Families of Pediatric Cochlear-Implant Candidate (2000)

When a Student Fails to Make the Grade (1999)

When Health Plans Limit Care (1996)

When Student and Supervisor Disagree about Patient Care (1998)

When Supervisors and Students Disagree (1998)

Note. From *American Speech-Language-Hearing Association Ethics Roundtable.* Retrieved May 12, 2006, from http://www.asha.org/about/ethics/roundtable.

acknowledging any research support, stating any financial relationship between authors and products, and listing any affiliations with direct interest in the subject (King, McGuire, Longman, & Carroll-Johnson, 1997).

Summary

The ASHA Code of Ethics has been revised several times because of expanded scopes of professional practice, expansion of client populations and practice settings, technological advances, and past ethical misconduct. The Code of Ethics provides guidelines that enable individuals to define ethical practice and standards against which potential violations can be considered. Failing to follow the Code of Ethics compromises professional services to clients, students, colleagues, and other professionals. There may be serious consequences for ethical misconduct, for example revocation of clinical certification and/or cancellation of ASHA membership. New ethical issues will continue to arise as professional practices evolve.

References

Ambrose, N. G., & Yairi, E. (2002). The Tudor Study: Data and ethics. *American Journal of Speech-Language Pathology, 11,* 190–203.

American Psychological Association (2001). *Publication manual of the American Psychological Association* (5th ed.). Washington, DC: Author.

American Speech and Hearing Association. (1952). Code of ethics of the American Speech and Hearing Association. *Journal of Speech and Hearing Disorders, 17,* 255–256.

American Speech and Hearing Association. (1965). Code of ethics of the American Speech and Hearing Association. *ASHA,* 230.

American Speech and Hearing Association. (1971). Code of ethics of the American Speech and Hearing Association. *ASHA,* 302.

American Speech and Hearing Association. (1975). Code of ethics of the American Speech and Hearing Association. *ASHA,* 58.

American Speech and Hearing Association. (1977). Code of ethics of the American Speech and Hearing Association. *ASHA,* 41–42.

American Speech and Hearing Association. (1979). Code of ethics of the American Speech and Hearing Association. *ASHA,* 25–26.

American Speech and Hearing Association. (1986, April). Code of ethics of the American Speech and Hearing Association. *ASHA,* 55–56.

American Speech and Hearing Association. (1990). Code of ethics of the American Speech and Hearing Association. *ASHA,* 37–38.

American Speech and Hearing Association. (1991). Code of ethics of the American Speech and Hearing Association. *ASHA,* 103–104.

American Speech and Hearing Association. (1992). *Code of ethics of the American Speech and Hearing Association.* Rockville, MD: Author.

American Speech-Language-Hearing Association. (1993). *Code of ethics.* Rockville, MD: Author.

American Speech-Language-Hearing Association. (1994, March). Code of ethics. *ASHA, 36*(Suppl. 13), 1–2.

American Speech-Language-Hearing Association. (2001a). Code of ethics. *ASHA Leader, 6*(23), 2–3.

American Speech-Language-Hearing Association. (2001b). Drawing cases for private practice from primary place of employment. *ASHA Supplement, 22,* 69–70.

American Speech-Language-Hearing Association. (2001c). Scope of practice in speech-language pathology. *ASHA Supplement, 22,* 29–36.

American Speech-Language-Hearing Association. (2001d). *Telepractices and ASHA.* Retrieved July 15, 2003, from http://search.asha.org/query.html?at-telepractice.

American Speech-Language-Hearing Association. (2001e). *Telepractices and ASHA: Report of the telepractices team.* Rockville, MD: Author.

American Speech-Language-Hearing Association. (2002). Ethics in research and professional practice. *ASHA Supplement, 22,* 63–65.

American Speech-Language-Hearing Association. (2003). Code of ethics. *ASHA Supplement, 22,* 13–15.

American Speech-Language-Hearing Association. (2004a). Admission/criteria in speech-language pathology. *ASHA Supplement, 24,* 65–70.

American Speech-Language-Hearing Association. (2004b). Conflicts of professional interest. *ASHA Supplement, 24,* 46–48.

American Speech-Language-Hearing Association. (2004b). Knowledge and skills needed by speech-language pathologists and audiologists to provide culturally and linguistically appropriate services. *ASHA Supplement, 24,* 152–158.

American Speech-Language-Hearing Association. (2004d). Scope of practice in audiology. *ASHA Supplement, 24,* 27–35.

American Speech-Language-Hearing Association. (2004e). Vocal tract visualization and imaging technical report. *ASHA Supplement, 24,* 140–145.

American Speech-Language-Hearing Association. (2005a). Cultural competence. *ASHA Supplement, 25.*

American Speech-Language-Hearing Association. (2005b). End-of-life issues. Retrieved from http://www.asha.org/members/s/p/clinical.

American Speech-Language-Hearing Association. (2005c). Speech-language pathologists providing clinical services via telepractice. Technical report. *ASHA Supplement.*

American Speech-Language-Hearing Association. (n.d.). *Commercialism/marketing policy.* Rockville, MD: Author.

Americans with Disabilities Act of 1990, Pub. L. No. 101–335, 2. 104 Stat. 328 (1991).

Annett, M. M. (2002). Article alleges 1939 study taught children to stutter. *ASHA Leader, 6*(13), 1, 17.

Blackmer, J. (2001). Tube feeding in stroke patients: A medical and ethical perspective. *Canadian Journal of Neurological Sciences, 28*(2), 101–106.

Bradley, S. B. (1995). Conflict of interest. In F. L. Macrina (Ed.), *Scientific integrity* (pp. 161–188). Washington, DC: ASM Press.

Canter, M. B., Bennett, B. E., Jones, S. E., & Nagy, T. F. (1999). *Ethics for psychologists.* Washington, DC: American Psychological Association.

Civil Rights Act of 1964, Pub. L. No. 88–352 (Title VII).

Denton, D. R. (2003). Ethical and legal issues related to telepractice. *Seminars in Speech and Language, 24*(4), 313–322.

Denton, D. R., & Gladstone, V. S. (2005). Ethical and legal issues related to telepractice. *Seminars in Hearing, 26*(1), 43–52.

Dyer, J. (2001, June 10). Ethics and orphans: The Monster study. Part one of a Mercury News Special Report. *San Jose [CA] Mercury News,* p. 1A.

Dyer, J. (2001, June 11). Ethics and orphans: The Monster study. Part two of a Mercury News Special Report. *San Jose [CA] Mercury News*, p. 1A.

Epstein, R. M., & Hundert, E. M. (2002). Defining and assessing professional competence. *Journal of the American Medical Association, 287*(2), 226–235.

Ernst, E., Cohen, M. H., & Stone, J. (2004). Ethical problems arising in evidence based complementary and alternative medicine. *Journal of Medical Ethics, 30*, 156–159.

Hamilton, N. W. (2002). *Academic ethics*. Westport, CT: Praeger Publishers.

Hawkins, D. B. (2000). Conflicts of interests and the audiologist. *Seminars in Hearing, 21*(1), 33–40.

Helm-Estabrooks, N. (2004). Forward: The times they are a-changin': Nontraditional treatment approaches to communication disorders. *Seminars in Speech and Language, 25*(2), 117–118.

Huffman, N. P. (2002, February 19). ASHA's Board of Ethics: Let's get acquainted. *ASHA Leader, 1*, 6–7.

Ingham, J. C. (2003). Research ethics 101: The responsible conduct of research. *Seminars in Speech and Language, 24*(4), 323–337.

Ingham, J. C., & Horner, J. (2004, March 16). Ethics and research. *ASHA Leader*, 10–11, 24–25.

Jacobson, G. P. (2002). Is the tail wagging the dog? *American Journal of Audiology,11*(1), 1–2.

Keith-Spiegel, P., Balogh, D. W., Whitley, B. E., Perkins, D. V., & Wittig, A. F. (2002). *The ethics of teaching*. Mahwah, NJ: Lawrence Erlbaum Associates.

King, C. R., McGuire, D. B., Longman, A. J., & Carroll-Johnson, R. M. (1997). Peer review, authorship, ethics, and conflict of interest. *Journal of Nursing Scholarship, 29*(2), 163–167.

King, D. (2003, May 22). Ethics supervision of student clinicians. *ASHA Leader*, 26.

Kirkwood, D. H. (2003). Survey of dispensers finds little consensus on what is ethical practice. *The Hearing Journal, 56*(3), 19–26.

Liang, B. A. (2000). Fraud and abuse in audiology: The law of conflict of interest. *Seminars in Hearing, 21*(1), 41–62.

Lo, B. (2003). Answers and questions about ethics consultations. *Journal of the American Medical Association, 290*(9), 1208–1210.

Lundgren, K. (2004). Preface: Complementary and alternative approaches to treating communication disorders. *Seminars in Speech and Language, 25*(2), 119–120.

McAllister, L., & Lincoln, M. (2004). *Clinical education in speech-language pathology.* London: Whurr Publishers.

McCartney, J. (2002, September 24). ASHA code of ethics and research. *ASHA Leader,* 12.

McCrea, E. S., & Brasseur, J. A. (2003). *The supervisory process in speech-language pathology.* Boston: Allyn & Bacon.

Meline, T., & Mata-Pistokache, T. (2003). The perils of Pauline's e-mail: Professional issues for audiologists and speech-language pathologists. *Contemporary Issues in Communication Sciences and Disorders, 30,* 118–122.

Metz, M. J. (2000). Some ethical issues related to hearing instrument dispensing. *Seminars in Hearing, 21*(1), 63–74.

Moxley, A., Mahendra, N., & Vega-Barachowitz, C. (2004, April 3). Cultural competence in health care. *ASHA Leader,* 6–7, 20–22.

Mustain, W. (2003, April 1). ASHA's code of ethics modified to address research ethics. *ASHA Leader,* 28.

National Society of Professional Engineers v. State of New York, 435 U.S. 679, 697–698 (1978).

Paden, E. P. (1970). *A history of the American Speech and Hearing Association 1925–1958.* Washington, DC: American Speech and Hearing Association.

Peach, R. K. (2003). From the editor. *American Journal of Speech-Language Pathology, 12,* 386.

Rao, P. R., & Martin, J. E. (2004, March 16). Treatment candidacy and ethical decision making. *ASHA Leader, 1,* 20–21.

Schneiderman, L. J., Gilmer, T., Teetzel, H. D., Dugan, D. O., Blustein, J., Crandordm, R., et al. (2003). Effect of ethics consultations on nonbeneficial life-sustaining treatments in the intensive care setting. *Journal of the American Medical Association, 290*(9), 1166–1172.

Sharp, H. M., & Bryant, K. M. (2003). Ethical issues in dysphagia. When patients refuse assessment or treatment. *Seminars in Speech and Language, 24*(4), 285–299.

Silverman, F. H. (1983). *Legal aspects of speech-language pathology and audiology.* Englewood Cliffs, NJ: Prentice Hall.

Sininger, Y., Marsh, R., Walden, B., & Wilber, L. A. (2003). Guidelines for ethical practice in research for audiologists. *Audiology Today, 15*(6), 14–17.

Strand, E. A., Yorkston, K. M., & Miller, R. M. (1998). Medical ethics and the speech-language pathologist. In A. F. Johnson & B. H. Jacobson (Eds.), *Medical speech-language pathology: A practitioner's guide* (pp. 192–210). New York: Thieme.

Strike, K. A., & Soltis, J. F. (1992). *The ethics of teaching.* New York: Teachers College Press.

Ulrich, S. R. (2004, November 2). Ethical considerations in patient discharge. *ASHA Leader,* 21–22.

Whicker, M. L., & Kronenfeld, J. J. (1994). *Dealing with ethical dilemmas on campus.* Thousands Oaks, CA: Sage.

Woltosz, W. D., Bristow, D. C., Fromkin, J. R., & Romich, B. (1994). The role of speech-language pathologists as manufacturers' representatives in ACC: Four opinions. *American Journal of Speech-Language Pathology, 3*(1), 11–18.

Chapter 3

Evolution of the AAA Code of Ethics

Learning Objectives

After reading this chapter, you should be able to:

- Discuss the evolution of the AAA Code of Ethics.
- Explain reasons for revision of the AAA's Code of Ethics.
- Identify current and future ethical issues related to audiology.
- Compare the AAA and ASHA codes.

Introduction

The Code of Ethics of the American Academy of Audiology ([AAA], 2003a) describes professional standards for audiologists. The Code has eight principles that are related to honesty and compassion, competence, confidentiality, best interest of persons served, accurate information, professionalism, public and professional responsibility, and ethical standards. Within each principle, there are specific rules of ethics. Appendix B provides an operational classification of these principles and rules.

 The First AAA Code of Ethics

The first Code of Ethics of the American Academy of Audiology was adopted in the fall of 1990 and published in January 1991 (Resnick, 1993). It consisted of two parts: (1) Statement of Principles and Rules, and (2) Procedures for the Management of Alleged Violations.

Revisions

There were minor changes in the 1996 revision of the Code of Ethics (AAA, 1996a). In 2003, there were major changes related to guidelines for ethical practice in research. These guidelines are listed in Table 3-1. One rule was eliminated: Rule 4d, which stated, "Individuals shall not accept compensation for supervision or sponsorship beyond reimbursement of expenses." This rule was eliminated because it prevented audiologists who supervise students from being compensated by the student's university (Sininger, Marsh, Walden, & Wilber, 2003). Compensation for supervision includes but is not limited to free continuing education activities and adjunct faculty benefits.

Table 3-1 AAA Code of Ethics: References to Research (AAA, 2003)

PRINCIPLE 1: Members shall provide professional services and conduct *research* with honesty and compassion, and shall respect the dignity, worth, and rights of those served.

> Rule 2c: Individuals shall exercise all reasonable precautions to avoid injury to persons in the delivery of professional services or execution of *research*.

PRINCIPLE 3: Members shall maintain the confidentiality of the information and records of those receiving services or involved in *research*.

> Rule 4d: Individuals using investigational procedures with patients, or prospectively collecting *research* data, shall first obtain full informed consent from the patient or guardian.

> Rule 5a: Individuals shall provide persons served with the information a reasonable person would want to know about the nature and possible effects of services rendered, or products provided or *research* being conducted.

> Rule 5c: Individuals shall conduct and report product-related research only according to accepted standards of *research* practice.

> Rule 5d: Individuals shall not carry out teaching or *research* activities in a manner that constitutes an invasion of privacy, or that fails to inform persons fully about the nature and possible effects of these activities, affording all persons informed free choice of participation.

> Rule 6b: Individuals' public statements about professional services, products, or *research* results shall not contain representations or claims that are false, misleading, or deceptive.

> Rule 7b: Individuals shall inform colleagues and the public in a manner consistent with the highest professional standards about products and services they have developed or *research* they have conducted.

 ## 2003 Codes of Ethics

The major changes in the 2003 Code of Ethics were related to research (AAA, 2003a). One principle and six rules were modified to include research and, as already noted, are listed in Table 3-1. One rule was added, which states: "Individuals using investigational procedures with patients or prospectively collecting research data, shall first obtain full informed consent from the patient's guardian."

In January 2005, the AAA Board of Ethics approved changes to Principle 2 and the addition of Rule 2a (J. M. Kukula, personal communication, June 19, 2005). The former was changed from "members shall maintain high professional competence in rendering services, providing only those professional services for which they are qualified by education and experience" to "members shall maintain high professional competence in rendering services" (AAA, 2003a). Rule 2a states, "Individuals shall provide only those professional services for which they are qualified by education and experience."

Issues in Ethics

Several ethical issues warrant discussion. These issues include the doctorate in audiology (AuD), competence, conflicts of interest, discrimination, misrepresentation, research, and telepractice. Obviously, these issues are evolving and will change over time.

Doctorate in Audiology

The professional doctorate in audiology (AuD) will be the entry-level degree for the profession by 2012 (AAA, 2005e; ASHA, 2005). The AuD typically requires four years of full-time study beyond the bachelor's degree. Steiger, Saccone, and Freeman (2002) proposed a doctor of audiology oath to affirm professionalism and ethical conduct.

Audiologists are divided about use of the title of doctor of audiology (Newman-Ryan, 2000). The AAA's Ethical Practices Board (AAAa, AAAb) has issued two advisory statements about the use of the term *doctor* in advertising and *AuD candidate*. *Doctor* alone is inappropriate; degree status must also be indicated, such as *PhD* or *AuD*. Public use of the term *AuD candidate* to indicate completion of the majority of the degree requirements is inappropriate.

Competence

The AAA Code of Ethics (AAA, 2003a) has one principle and three rules related to **competence.** Principle 2 addresses "high standards of professional competence." The rules address delegating services only to competent persons (2e); maintaining professional competence, such as by continuing education (2g); and public statements about competence (6b).

Conflicts of Interest

The AAA Code of Ethics (AAA, 2003a), Rule 4c, indicates, "Individuals shall not participate in activities that constitute a conflict of professional interest." Hawkins (2000) believes the AAA Code of Ethics should be more precise and provide specific guidelines about conflicts of interest. According to Liang (2000), "some common financial arrangements in the field have strayed dangerously close to violating the laws of fraud and abuse" (p. 41).

The Academy's Ethical Practices Board (AAA, 1997) described **conflict of interest** as including all activities related to the practice of audiology in which professional decisions could be compromised. The board (AAA, 2003b) further defined *conflict of interest* in ethical guidelines on financial incentives from hearing instrument manufacturers. It was stated that "any gifts accepted by the audiologist should principally benefit the patient and should not be of substantial value (< $100)." Furthermore, "audiologists should not participate in any industry sponsored social function that may appear to bias professional judgment or practices." This includes invitations to private convention parties or golf outings or accepting items such as theater tickets. Meals and social events that are part of an educational program are acceptable. The Ethical Guidelines also provide answers for the fifteen most frequently asked questions about financial incentives from hearing instrument manufacturers. The board has also issued three advisory statements related to conflict of interest: (1) "Buying groups, rewards, and conflicts of interest" (AAA, 2004a); (2) "Buying groups, trips, cash rebates and conflicts of interest" (AAA, 2004b); and "To party, or not to party? That is the question" (2004c).

Metz (2000) described hearing aid dispensing and pointed out that high ethical standards and good business decisions are difficult because "professional and business perceptions and goals are many times in conflict on a basic level." Furthermore, because there are few absolutes related to ethics, there is little consensus as to what is ethical practice (Metz, 2000). Two surveys of professional activities found little agreement about areas of potential conflicts of interest. One survey (Hawkins, Hamill, Van Vliet, & Freeman, 2002) included 182 audiologists and 42 adults with hearing impairment. The other survey (Kirkwood, 2003) was of 600 audiologists, hearing aid dealers, and otolaryngologists.

Audiologists should be aware of potential conflicts of interest. Avoiding conflicts of interest involves an awareness of potential conflicts. Hawkins (2000) described several areas of potential conflicts of interest: commercial interest in a hearing aid company; social relationships with commercial enterprises; and rebates, gifts, and awards for products dispensed. Jacobson (2002) identified several conflicts related to industry such as support of graduate students, development of dispensing practices, presentations at national professional meetings, continuing education outside national meetings, development funds, and partnership points.

Discrimination
There is specific reference to **discrimination** in the AAA Code of Ethics (AAA, 2003a). Principle 2, Rule 2d states, "Individuals . . . shall not discriminate in the provision of services to individuals on the basis of sex, race, religion, national origin, sexual orientation, or general health."

Misrepresentation
The current AAA Code of Ethics (AAA, 2003a) has four provisions related to misrepresentation, that is, misleading or misinforming. Rules addressing this issue are related to prognosis (5b); professional training and experience (6a);

public statements about services, products, or research results (6b); and professional or commercial affiliation (7a).

Research

Audiologists may be involved in activities that are not usually considered as research but that involve many of the same ethical issues (Sininger et al., 2003). These are issues related to authorship in publication and presentation of research, adequacy of research design and protection of data, and conflict of interest in product-oriented outcomes of research. Guidelines related to these issues were discussed by Sininger et al. (2003).

It should be noted that the AAA Code of Ethics (AAA, 2003a) was modified to address research ethics but does not specifically mention authorship or referencing of sources. The Research Committee of the AAA (2005c, 2005d) has guidelines for research and publication that should help audiologists and others maintain ethical standards in research.

Telepractice

The use of **telepractice** in audiology resulted from changes in practice patterns, the need to provide services long distance to underserved populations, and innovations in technology (Elangovan, 2005; Krumm, Ribera, & Schmiedge, 2005; Ribera, 2005; Towers, Pisa, Froelich, & Krumm, 2005; Waguespack, 2005. Yates & Campbell, 2005). There is no specific reference to telepractice in the AAA Code of Ethics (AAA, 2003a), although there are several standards related to telepractice. These standards include **competence** (Principle 2), use of support personnel (Rules 2d), informed consent (Rule 4d), and privacy and confidentiality (Principle 3, Rule 3a).

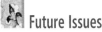 Future Issues

Helmick (2000) believes that audiology will be challenged in the future by "... the degree to which the profession of audiology is merged with the business of audiology"

Table 3-2 AAA Guidelines and Advisories

Buying groups, rewards, and conflicts of interest (AAA, 2004a)

Buying groups, trips, cash rebates, and conflicts of interest (AAA, 2004b)

Ethical practice guidelines on financial incentives from hearing instrument manufacturers (AAA, 2003b)

Guidelines on conflicts of interest (AAA, 1997)

Guidelines for ethical practice in research for audiologists (Sininger et al., 2003)

"To party, or not to party? That is the question." (AAA, 2004c)

Use of the term *AuD candidate* (AAA, 2005a)

Use of the term *Doctor* advertising (AAA, 2005b)

(p. 47). Other issues are related to (1) ensuring competency in the context of an expanding scope of practice, (2) balancing service and business, and (3) identifying and establishing guidelines for conflicts of interest.

AAA's Ethical Guidelines and Advisories

The AAA periodically provides guidelines and advisories to increase awareness of the Academy's Code of Ethics and the practical application of the ethical principles and rules. These guidelines and advisories are listed in Table 3-2. Recently, the AAA published a book devoted to ethics, *Ethics in Audiology; Guidelines for Ethical Conduct in Clinical, Educational, and Research Settings* (AAA, 2006).

Comparison of AAA and ASHA Codes of Ethics

There appear to be more similarities than differences in the AAA and ASHA codes of ethics. The content of these codes is remarkably similar (Newman-Ryan & Decker, 2000). The ethical codes of AAA and ASHA both seek to promote similar values (Helmick, 2000). Each code cites as its first and highest ethical principle the responsibility to consider the "benefit" (AAA, 2003a) and "welfare" (ASHA, 2003) of those served professionally. Additional comparisons of the two codes are presented in Table 3-3. Another similarity is that both AAA (1996b) and ASHA (2001, 2004) have Scope of Practice statements.

Table 3-3 Comparison of AAA and ASHA Codes of Ethics

	AAA	ASHA
First Code	1991	1930
Year Organized	1988	1925
Signature Required	Yes	No
Members	Audiologists	Speech-language pathologists Audiologists
Board	Ethical Practices Board	Board of Ethics
Latest Revision	2003	2003
Principles	8	4
Rules	26	37
Parts	2: Principles and Rules; Procedures for Violations	1: Principles and Rules
Doctorate	Use of terms *Doctor* and *AuD candidate*	_____

Both codes address issues related to confidentiality, discrimination, competence, referrals, prognosis, supervision, conflict of interest, and informing and complying with the academy and/or the association about ethical misconduct. Research and scholarly activities were expanded in the revisions of both codes. The AAA Code of Ethics has specific rules related to avoiding injury (2c), exploitation of persons served (4a), product-oriented research (5c), and invasion of privacy (5d). The AAA, unlike ASHA, has no specific provisions related to maintenance of equipment (II-F), autonomy (Principle IV), substance abuse (I-O), sexual misconduct (IV-C), publication credit or authorship (IV-D), referencing sources (IV-E), and telepractice (I-J).

Confidentiality is both an ethical and a legal issue (Aiken, 2002). Both ASHA's Code of Ethics (Principle I, Rule L) and AAA's Code of Ethics (Principle 3) address confidentiality. The Health Insurance Portability and Accountability Act (HIPAA) established federal standards for release of information including privacy of protected health information, transmission of electronic data, and security of data (Golper & Brown, 2004). Both codes of ethics and HIPAA emphasize the client's right to confidentiality of information in their records.

HIPAA regulations apply to any aspects of health care services that involve transmission of any related information in an electronic form or database. The transmission of all health care information (oral, written, or fax) and the maintenance of electronic and paper records are covered by HIPAA. The law permits disclosure of information about treatment, payment for services, and health care operations. Failure to comply with HIPAA regulations can result in penalties including fines and even imprisonment.

Summary

The AAA is a professional organization for audiologists that has a Code of Ethics and ethical guidelines about a variety of topics. There are several critical ethical issues for audiologists. These issues include but are not limited to competence, conflicts of interest, discrimination, misrepresentation, research, and telepractice. This chapter also presented a comparison of the AAA and ASHA codes of ethics.

References

Aiken, T. D. (2002). *Legal and ethical issues in health occupations.* Philadelphia: W. B. Saunders.

American Academy of Audiology. (1996a). *Code of ethics and procedures, rules, and penalties.* Ruston, VA: Author.

American Academy of Audiology. (1996b). *Scope of practice in audiology.* Ruston, VA: Author.

American Academy of Audiology. (1997, March/April). Issues in ethics: Conflicts of professional interests. *Audiology Today, 26.*

American Academy of Audiology. (2003a). *Code of ethics and procedures, rules, and penalties.* Retrieved from http://www.audiology.org/professional/ethics.

American Academy of Audiology. (2003b). Ethical practice guidelines on financial incentives from hearing instrument manufacturers. *Audiology Today, 15*(3), 19–21.

American Academy of Audiology. (2004a). Buying groups, rewards, and conflicts of interest. *Audiology Today, 16*(3), 28.

American Academy of Audiology. (2004b). Ethical Practices Board: Buying groups, trips, cash rebates, and conflicts of interest. *Audiology Today, 16*(1), 9.

American Academy of Audiology. (2004c). Ethical Practices Board: To party, or not to party? That is the question. *Audiology Today, 16*(2), 43.

American Academy of Audiology. (2005b). *Ethical Practice Board advisory statement on the term "AuD candidate."* Retrieved from http://www.audiology.org/professional/ethics/adv-aud.php.

American Academy of Audiology. (2005c). *Ethical Practice Board advisory statement on use of the term "doctor" in advertising.* Retrieved from http://www.audiology.org/professional/ethics/adv-doctor.php.

American Academy of Audiology. (2005d). *FAQs for publishing.* Retrieved May 23, 2005, from http://www.audiology.org/students/research/pubfaq.php.

American Academy of Audiology. (2005e). *FAQs for undertaking a research project.* Retrieved May 23, 2005, from http://www.audiology.org/students/research/rpfaq.php.

American Academy of Audiology. (2005f). *What you need to know about the AuD degree.* Retrieved May 18, 2005, from http://www.audiology.org/students/audfacts.php.

American Academy of Audiology. (2006). *Ethics in audiology: Guidelines for ethical conduct in clinical, educational, and research settings.* Ruston, VA: Author.

American Speech-Language-Hearing Association. (2001). *Scope of practice in speech-language pathology.* Rockville, MD: Author.

American Speech-Language-Hearing Association. (2003). Code of ethics. *ASHA Supplement, 23,* 12–15.

American Speech-Language-Hearing Association. (2004). Scope of practice in audiology. *ASHA Supplement, 24,* 27–35.

American Speech-Language-Hearing Association. (2005). *New audiology standards.* Retrieved from http://www.asha.org/about/membershipcertification/certification/aud_standards_new.htm.

Elangovan, S. (2005). Telehearing and the Internet. *Seminars in Hearing, 26*(1), 19–25.

Golper, L. A., & Brown, J. E. (2004). *Business matters: A guide for speech-language pathologists.* Rockville, MD: American Speech-Language-Hearing Association.

Hawkins, D. B. (2000). Conflicts of interest and the audiologist. *Seminars in Hearing, 21*(1), 33–40.

Hawkins, D. E., Hamill, T., Van Vliet, D., & Freeman, B. (2002). Potential conflicts of interest as viewed by the audiologist and the hearing-impaired consumer. *Audiology Today, 14*(5), 27–32.

Helmick, J. W. (2000). Professional ethics and audiology. In H. Hosford-Dunn, R. J. Roeser, and L. M. Valente (Eds.), *Audiology practice management* (pp. 41–48). New York: Thieme.

Jacobson, G. P. (2002). "Is the tail wagging the dog?" *American Journal of Audiology, 11*(1), 2–3.

Kirkwood, D. H. (2003). Survey of dispensers finds little consensus on what is ethical practice. *Hearing Journal, 56*(3), 19–26.

Krumm, M., Ribera, J., & Schmiedge, J. (2005). Using a telehealth medium for objective hearing testing: Implications for supporting rural universal newborn hearing screening programs. *Seminars in Hearing, 26*(1), 3–12.

Liang, B. A. (2000). Fraud and abuse in audiology: The law of conflict of interest. *Seminars in Hearing, 21*(1), 41–62.

Metz, M. J. (2000). Some ethical issues related to hearing instrument dispensing. *Seminars in Hearing, 21*(1), 63–74.

Newman-Ryan, J. (2000). History of professional health care ethics. *Seminars in Hearing, 21*(1), 3–20.

Newman-Ryan, J., & Decker, T. N. (2000). Ethics in professional practice. In H. Hosford-Dunn, R. J. Roeser, & M. Valente (Eds.), *Audiology practice management* (pp. 207–230). New York: Thieme.

Resnick, D. M. (1993). *Professional ethics for audiologists and speech-language pathologists.* Clifton Park, NY: Thomson Delmar Learning.

Ribera, J. E. (2005). Interjudge reliability and validation of telehealth applications of the hearing in noise test. *Seminars in Hearing, 26*(1), 13–18.

Sininger, Y., Marsh, R., Walden, B., & Wilber, L. A. (2003). Guidelines for ethical practice on research for audiologists. *Audiology Today, 15*(6), 14–17.

Steiger, J., Saccone, P. A., & Freeman, (2002). A proposed doctoral oath for audiologists. *Audiology Today, 14*(6), 12–14.

Towers, A. D., Pisa, J., Froelich, T. M., & Krumm, M. (2005). The reliability of click-evoked and frequency-specific auditory brain stem response testing using telehealth technology. *Seminars in Hearing, 26*(1), 26–34.

Waguespack, G. M. (2005). The regulation of telepractice in the profession of audiology. *Seminars in Hearing, 26*(1), 53–55.

Yates, J. T., & Campbell, I. H. (2005). Audiovestibular education and services via telemedicine technologies. *Seminars in Hearing, 26*(1), 35–42.

Chapter 4

Ethical Decision Making

Learning Objectives

After reading this chapter, you should be able to:

- Discuss the personal values and beliefs that influence ethical decision making.
- Describe six steps used for ethical decision making.
- Apply case scenarios for speech-language pathology and audiology utilizing an ethical decision-making model.
- Describe options for reporting alleged ethical violations.
- Discuss enforcement for alleged ethical violations by a variety of boards, agencies, or organizations.

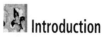 Introduction

The process of making ethical decisions involves a multitude of factors and experiences. These factors can include but are not limited to personal beliefs, moral values, laws and regulations, number of years of experience in the profession, the outcomes of previous decisions, and client and/or family issues/preferences. Any professional making ethical decisions should adopt and/or develop a logical process that includes steps that can lead to positive outcomes for the benefit of all involved. This chapter provides a model for ethical decision making that can be used to guide the process. In addition, there is information in this chapter that provides suggestions for reporting and enforcing of ethical rules and principles that are used by professional organizations and/or licensure boards.

The Steps in Ethical Decision Making

Ethical decision making should involve a sequence of logical steps that will support the professional. Decision-making models in ethics are used by various health professions (Chabon & Morris, 2004; Gabard & Martin, 2003; Harman, 2001; Kilmas, 2001; Purtilo, 1999; Weinstein, 2001). Common steps can be identified from these practicing models to help guide professionals and future speech-language pathologists (SLPs) and audiologists (AUDs) through the process of making decisions, resulting in resolution of an ethical dilemma.

External and Internal Factors

Figure 4-1 depicts a model that involves ethical decision making that is both logical and practical. The model begins by listing a variety of external and internal factors that are relevant to the specific situation. These external factors may include job responsibilities, prognosis of the client, wishes and needs of the client/family, and employment-setting policies. Internal factors may include personal values and beliefs of the professional, past

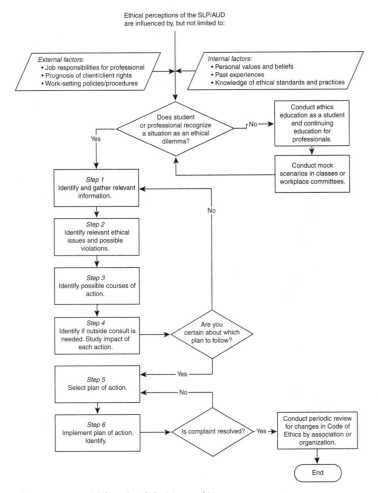

Figure 4-1 Model for ethical decision making.

clinical experiences, education and knowledge of clinical skills, and knowledge of ethical standards and practice.

Does the Clinician Recognize an Ethical Dilemma?

In Figure 4-1, the ethical decision-making model includes an important question: Does the clinician recognize a situation as an ethical dilemma? Although most individuals will probably respond "yes" to this question, it is important that the situation be clearly defined and that it address relevant professional issues. If the answer is "no," then steps should be taken to educate oneself and to clarify the issue. Current ASHA certification standards require documentation of ethical knowledge and adherence to the ASHA Code of Ethics in speech-language pathology and audiology (ASHA, 2005a, 2005b). Demonstrating knowledge of a code of ethics upon graduation does not necessarily mean that the practicing professional will continue to know, understand, interpret, and apply the current code of ethics for a particular organization. As noted earlier in this book, the codes of ethics for ASHA, AAA, and many licensing boards have changed as the scope of practice changes.

Case-based scenarios have been used to understand how ethical dilemmas may be addressed and resolved (Purtilo, 1999). Case scenarios should be a method of instruction at both the undergraduate and graduate levels. Harman (2001) encourages ethics education and case-based scenarios so a clinician can make more reliable judgments and improve reasoning skills. Committees in employment settings are charged with the development and implementation of numerous policies and procedures in schools, hospitals, health care companies, and universities. The members of ethics or code of conduct committees should consider the discussion of mock or real-life, case-based scenarios to help clarify and prevent ethical dilemmas (Pannbacker & Irwin, 2003). Furthermore, it is important that the steps involved in ethical decision making be clear and allow for application and flexibility to numerous situations. Professional associations and organizations should encourage and/or sponsor discussions of ethical scenarios that will allow professionals to obtain mandatory continuing education units (CEUs) and also help improve clinical practice across all work settings (Kilmas, 2001).

Step 1: Identify and Gather Relevant Information.
Step 1 in Figure 4-1 involves the identification and gathering of relevant information regarding an **ethical dilemma.**

This step requires that the clinician focus upon the pertinent issues and not be "distracted" by other issues (e.g., personal issues such as a poor working relationship with a supervisor or personality conflicts with a parent). Fact gathering includes providing appropriate documentation, as well as identifying and possibly meeting with all interested parties. Chabon and Morris (2004) contend that "many ethical dilemmas originate from a lack of all the facts and values involved in a given situation, or from the failure to clearly explicate the problem" (p. 18). The **ethics boards** for ASHA and AAA require that the complainant provide written factual information before an allegation can be considered (ASHA, 2002; AAA, 2003). Pannbacker (1998) states that reporting an ethical violation is a "difficult ethical dilemma" and cautions any complainant or accuser against including facts that are not relevant or that may be viewed as personally vindictive.

For Case Scenario 4-1 and Case Scenario 4-2, please address how the professional would approach completing Step 1 in the decision-making model shown in Figure 4-1.

CASE SCENARIO 4-1

> A supervisor is concerned about the accuracy of a graduate student's phonetic transcription, which could result in inaccurate information being used and possibly resulting in an incorrect diagnosis.

Questions for Case Scenario 4-1 include: Which information is important to gather about this situation? Is this an ethical dilemma for only the supervisor? What are the facts? Which facts are most relevant?

Any inquiry about a possible ethical dilemma must be investigated with a review of what is known and unknown about the situation. The following facts are known in Case Scenario 4-1:

- Accuracy of the student's phonetic transcription may or may not be adequate.

- The supervisor is concerned about transcription adequacy.

- Transcription errors could compromise quality of services.
- Transcription adequacy can be evaluated objectively.

The following facts are unknown in Case Scenario 4-1:

- How accurate are the transcriptions?
- What is the nature of the client's disorder (e.g., structural anomalies)?
- Is the diagnosis consistent with the data?
- Does either transcriber have a hearing disorder?
- How well did the student perform in relevant courses (e.g., phonetics)?
- Has transcription accuracy been questioned by other supervisors?
- How can the accuracy of these transcriptions be improved?
- What type of professional development will expand the scope of competence?

The facts that are unknown about the situation could be addressed by collecting data such as tape recordings, student and supervisor transcriptions, audiograms from hearing tests of supervisor and student, and instrumental measures such as waveform and spectrographic measures. Analysis of these data would include interjudge agreement (supervisor and student), instrumental analysis, review of previous skills and outcomes for the students, and previous supervision strategies used by other faculty if phonetic transcription was noted as a concern.

Does an ethical dilemma only exist for the clinical supervisor? No, because the student should have concern about the welfare of the client (Principle I of ASHA) and competence (Principle II of ASHA).

Case Scenario 4-2

An audiologist, who is a member of AAA and is ASHA certified, is asked by a hearing aid vendor to accept $400 for each digital hearing aid that is sold.

In Case Scenario 4-2, the professional must identify and gather relevant information and ask questions such as, but not limited to, the following: Who is involved in this ethical dilemma? How should the AUD proceed with the collection of facts? Which facts are most relevant?

The following facts are known in Case Scenario 4-2:

- The AUD is a certified member of ASHA and AAA and is bound by the code of ethics for each organization.
- The hearing aid vendor offers $400 for each digital hearing aid that is sold.
- Digital hearing aids are generally more expensive for the public.
- Digital technology benefits some (not all) clients.

The following facts are unknown about the situation:

- What are the characteristics and functional needs of the clients?
- How do the specifications of these digital hearing aids compare with other options?
- What are the details of the vendor's offer? Contract? Stipulations? Quota?
- Does the vendor's offer impact the cost to the end user?
- Has the audiologist agreed to accept the vendor's offer?

The AUD and the hearing aid vendor are directly involved, and clients could be indirectly involved in this dilemma. The AUD reviews the ASHA Code of Ethics and notes that ASHA Principle I (welfare of clients), ASHA Principle III (responsibility to the public), AAA Principle 1 (honesty, compassion, respect), AAA Principle 4 (best interest of those served), and AAA Principle 7 (responsibility to the public) are relevant.

The AUD should proceed with the collection of facts by reviewing the written agreement or contract of the vendor, the specifications and characteristics of the hearing aid, and the audiological assessment of clients being considered for the fitting of the hearing aid.

The information found in Step 1 can be very useful when determining if further action is necessary, ethical, and in the best interest of all parties involved. Fact gathering should continue throughout the decision-making process as new situations and/or variables relevant to the case arise.

Step 2: Identify Relevant Ethical Issues and Possible Violations.

During Step 2, one must identify the relevant ethical issues and possible violations. The general principles of ethics (autonomy, beneficence, justice, and nonmaleficence, as presented in Chapter 1) and rules (ASHA, AAA, etc.) are reviewed in the context of the codes of ethics and practice standards. After one reviews the factual information, it is possible that what was originally thought to be a violation was not, in fact, a transgression or perhaps was presented with misinformation to all interested parties. When facts and relevant materials are obtained, the complainant should carefully review all principles and rules. Discussion with a colleague or an ethics consultant (without compromising confidentiality) may take place and help one to determine whether a violation exists (Pannbacker, 1998). It is recommended that a complainant review publications (within and outside the professions) for similar cases and determine potential violations (Harman, 2001; Gabard & Martin, 2003; Purtilo, 1999).

Utilize Case Scenario 4-3 to discuss how Step 2 of the ethical decision-making model may be applied.

CASE SCENARIO 4-3

A speech-language pathologist is employed as a clinical fellow (CF) by a health care company that serves nursing homes. The SLP-CF is relatively inexperienced and asks the supervisor to help with the identification of clients in need of speech-language services. While the SLP-CF is not at work one day, the supervisor comes to the nursing home and identifies several clients at the nursing home and leaves a written note to initiate treatment. When the SLP-CF

CASE SCENARIO 4-3 *(continued)* ▬▬▬▬▬▬▬▬▬▬▬▬

initiates treatment to the clients, it is discovered that several of the clients are not good candidates for treatment and are unlikely to benefit from services. When the SLP-CF calls the supervisor and says that several of the clients are unlikely to benefit from services, the supervisor for the CF responds that there is a "quota" of billable hours per week and that these clients must be served for the SLP-CF to maintain employment.

These are the questions for Case Scenario 4-3: What are the relevant ethical issues? What are the possible violations? What information must be gathered? What information is most relevant?

Utilizing Step 1, it is important to first determine which facts are known or unknown about the situation. Facts that are known include:

• The SLP-CF has limited experience and works in the nursing home.

• The supervisor identifies potential clients and asks the SLP-CF to initiate treatment.

• The SLP-CF initiates treatment and questions potential benefit to clients.

• The supervisor requires a "quota" for CF to retain employment.

It is also important to review which facts are unknown:

• What is the nature of the clients' impairment?

• What factors limit the clients' prognosis?

• Are the supervisor's referrals to enhance clients' welfare?

• Does the CF possess adequate skills, knowledge, and judgment?

• Is the CF's concern about potential benefit well founded?

• Is communication between the CF and the supervisor adequate?

- Are the billable hours or is the "quota" requirement in writing?
- Was the CF knowledgeable about this requirement when employed?

The CF reviews the ASHA Code of Ethics and determines that possible violations include ASHA Principle I (welfare of clients), ASHA Principle II (professional competence), ASHA Principle III (responsibility to the public) and the ASHA Principle I, Rule A (provide all service competently), ASHA Principle I, Rule E (delegate appropriately), ASHA Principle I, Rule G (provide services only if benefit is expected), ASHA Principle II, Rule D (delegate appropriately), and ASHA Principle III, Rule C (refer in clients' best interest and not based on personal finances).

Information that must be gathered includes:

- Interviews with clients and significant others to determine need/benefit
- Behavioral observation of clients
- Standardized assessment of clients
- Informal assessment of clients
- Billable hours requirement (e.g., written or implied?)
- Documentation by supervisor as to how needs of clients were determined

The CF should analyze the strengths and needs of each client, review what prerequisite skills are needed to determine the presence of communication disorders in this population, and analyze whether there are limitations in the knowledge and skills for the CF and/or the CF supervisor.

Step 3: Identify Possible Courses of Action.

Identification of one's possible courses of action is the third step of the model. Utilizing information from Step 1 and Step 2, one must consider which of several possible courses of action may be the best. Oftentimes, Step 3 involves a series of "gray" questions/answers and ethical conflicts. This step includes but is not limited to legal issues; regulatory (licensure/certification) rules; and impact upon the client, employee, employer, and public perception of the professions (Chabon & Morris, 2004).

Using Case Scenario 4-4, apply Step 3 in the ethical decision-making model depicted in Figure 4-1.

CASE SCENARIO 4-4

An audiologist is employed at a large regional hospital. The AUD is testing the success of three different types of digital hearing aids from a company. The AUD wants a client to be involved as a participant, but the study has not been approved by the Institutional Review Board (IRB) at the hospital. The AUD decides to have the client try the various hearing aids and thinks the IRB will approve the study anyway. The AUD does disclose to the client that he is part of a research study. The AUD decides not to charge the client for services and asks him to not tell anyone about it.

The questions for Case Scenario 4-4 follow: What are the possible courses of action that should be considered by the AUD? Are there issues about legal action, ethical decisions, or honesty? If so, define and discuss these items and provide possible courses of action by the AUD who is licensed by the state, is certified by ASHA, and is a member of AAA and ASHA.

Prior to this step, it is assumed that the AUD has already conducted Step 1 and Step 2, which primarily involve fact gathering and considering which ethical violations might be involved. What would you do during Step 1 and Step 2? What led you to those decisions for Step 1 and Step 2? Now, the following data should be collected by the AUD in this scenario to use when considering possible courses of action:

• Review of research guidelines and IRB documentation
• List of potential risks/benefits

- Results of client's audiogram
- Hearing aid specifications
- Client's comments about the interaction and the request by the AUD to not let others know (obtained during client interview)

Possible courses of action are:

- The AUD must obtain IRB approval.
- The AUD must discuss resolution with the client (the client has a negative reaction about the lack of written informed consent and about misrepresentation).
- The client may file a grievance with the hospital committee.

All possible courses of action should be carefully considered. Depending on the type of action taken, it could drive the type of legal, ethical, or moral issues involved with the clinical issue. "Pilot studies" are usually done while clarifying procedures and are sometimes exempt from IRB approval. In this particular scenario, what if the AUD tells the client that his intention was to "pilot" the use of the three hearing aids and did not obtain IRB approval for that reason?

Step 4: Identify Need for Outside Consultation and Impact If Outside Consultation Needed; Study Impact of Each Action.

Step 4 involves the evaluation of the necessity of consultation with someone who is not a part of the ethical dilemma. This may have occurred in a less formal manner during Step 2 (i.e., identifying relevant ethical issues and possible violations). Discussion with an ethics consultant (e.g., a colleague from a previous employer or a professor) may enhance one's ability to be objective and fair. Students may turn to a faculty supervisor or other colleagues. Consultation with someone who is a member of a board of ethics (i.e., ASHA, AAA, state licensing, state association) in another employment setting also may provide a unique perspective. Legal counsel, free or hired, may be the best course of action, particularly when the allegations are of a very serious nature and could involve criminal acts by the professional. The professional seeking advice must fully understand and carefully evaluate the impact of any action being contemplated. For example, if the action is to report a supervisor to the company's Rules and Ethics Committee, then what will be the impact? Who will be affected? Will services for clients be compromised? What is the desired outcome or result? What are the complainant's motives for reporting the alleged ethical violation? If the professional and/or student cannot make a decision about which plan of action to pursue, then it is important that Step 1 through Step 3 be repeated. Chabon and Morris (2004) suggest the use of a consensus model, which "is agreement to proceed in a certain way. It is not 100% unanimity, nor is it a compromise, understood in the typical sense of each party giving up values and beliefs to reach agreement" (p. 18).

Using Case Scenario 4-5, discuss how the professional may proceed and the possible courses of action. Can a consensus be achieved as described by Chabon and Morris?

CASE SCENARIO 4-5

An SLP, Maria, who is a certified member of ASHA and licensed by the state, works as an employee in a private practice. Maria suspects that her supervisor and owner of the private practice, Nicole, is billing for time during which no direct client service is provided (e.g., while writing plans of care). Nicole is a certified member of ASHA and also licensed by the state. Maria has a good friend in the billing office of the practice, Charlene. During a conversation, Maria confides in Charlene about Nicole's billing for services. Maria is told by Charlene that this is occurring and they agree that this is a violation of billing for services that are not rendered. The possible courses of action being considered by Maria are: (1) to confront Nicole and ask that it not occur again, (2) to report Nicole to the Legal Affairs Department of Medicare and other third-party payors, and (3) to report Nicole to the ASHA Board of Ethics and the State Licensure Board for Speech-Language Pathology and Audiology.

Has Maria completed the necessary steps to act? To address this question, the facts of what is known and unknown should be reviewed. The known facts are:

- ASHA-certified SLPs are bound by the Code of Ethics and state licensure laws.
- Maria suspects that her supervisor bills for indirect services.
- Maria discusses and confirms her suspicion with the billing representative.
- Maria considers three courses of action:
  - Confront supervisor, Nicole, and request this type of billing not occur again.
  - Report Nicole to the legal affairs office of payors.
  - Report Nicole to ASHA's Board of Ethics and the State Licensure Board for Speech-Language Pathology and Audiology.

The unanswered questions are:

- Is there written evidence that Nicole is billing inappropriately?
- Do certain payors allow for reimbursement of indirect client service?
- How will legal affairs offices of payors respond to a complaint?
- How will ASHA and the State Licensure Board respond to a complaint?
- How will Nicole respond when Maria talks with her about her concern?
- What is the potential impact of any course of action upon client welfare?

In addition, Maria should review the codes of ethics for ASHA and the State Board of Examiners for Speech-Language Pathologists. In this instance, the state licensure laws and rules of ethics are very similar to those of ASHA's Board of Ethics. Maria determines that the following ASHA Principles of Ethics could be violated: Principle I: client welfare; Principle III: responsibility to the public;

and Principle IV: responsibility to the profession. Potentially the following Rules of Ethics may be violated: ASHA Principle I, Rule M: possible misrepresentation of services; ASHA Principle III, Rule D: prohibits misrepresentation and fraud; ASHA Principle IV, Rule F: prohibits misrepresentation to colleagues; ASHA Principle IV, Rule I: requires reporting of ethical violations; and ASHA Principle IV, Rule J: requires compliance with ethical board.

What are the possible outcomes of the actions being considered by Maria?

- Maria confronts Nicole about her suspicion in a private meeting. Nicole becomes angry and asks Maria the reasons behind her allegations and states that all records for her clients are confidential and would violate HIPAA if she allowed Maria to see them. At this point, should Maria report Nicole to a regulatory board or agency? If Maria does report Nicole and it is determined there are serious violations that could close the practice, what would happen to the clients?

- Nicole realizes that she has been doing something that is questionable and tells Maria that it will not happen again. Maria accepts Nicole's promise to not do this again. How would she monitor whether Nicole complied?

- Nicole accepts the responsibility for her actions and notifies third-party payors that refunds will be issued. Because she has agreed to pay restitution to the third-party payors, she is given a verbal warning by all third-party payors and all refunds are completed. Nicole is allowed to continue to practice. How will this action be monitored? Should Charlene in billing be the person to monitor this?

Step 5: Select Plan of Action.
Step 5 involves the selection of a plan of action. Selection of a plan can be a very difficult step in the decision-making process because it will involve some type of conflict with the alleged violator (parent, family member, other professional, student). However, if Step 1 through

Step 4 have been completed correctly and are supported by documented evidence, the complainant should be confident in going through with the plan of action. If not, the complainant can repeat Step 1 through Step 4 again to be more certain. Taking a "wait and see" attitude about the situation does not mean that it will be resolved on its own or get less complicated. The individual (complainant) has the obligation to report ethical misconduct to the appropriate supervisor (as specified in a code of conduct), committee(s), board(s), and/or organization(s) (Harman, 2001; Juengst, 1999; Pannbacker, 1998).

In Case Scenario 4-5, who should receive the alleged violation from Maria? Would it have to be sent to a particular board or organization? Two possible plans of action follow:

- Maria reports Nicole to the Legal Affairs Department of Medicare. The Legal Affairs Department requires Maria to sign a Waiver of Confidentiality that will mean that her identity will be known by Nicole. The Legal Affairs Department proceeds with its investigation and subpoenas Nicole's clinical records. If Medicare determines that serious violations did occur, Nicole may be reprimanded, pay fines, and be banned from serving Medicare clients. This outcome could lead to the closure of Nicole's private practice. In addition, Medicare informs the Board of Ethics of ASHA and also the State Board of Examiners for Speech-Language Pathology and Audiology. These boards concur with the findings of Medicare and revoke Nicole's CCC and state license. Nicole becomes very upset with Maria and threatens retaliation. Maria consults with an attorney about what protections she has from retaliation.

- Maria reports to the ASHA Board of Ethics and the State Board of Examiners for Speech-Language Pathology and Audiology. ASHA and the State Board of Examiners for Speech-Language Pathology and Audiology require Maria to sign a Waiver of Confidentiality. Following an investigation, the Board of Ethics for each organization determines that Nicole did not commit any ethical violations. Because no violations were found, these boards do not feel that this would need to be reported to Medicare. Nicole is upset with Maria and asks why she did not ask her before contacting an outside board. Nicole does not relieve Maria of her job.

Step 6: Implement Plan of Action.

Step 6 involves the implementation of a plan of action. This step requires that the professional reporting the alleged ethical violation be prepared to present factual and relevant information. Face-to-face discussions with the alleged violator or other relevant individuals will be a part of the process. Unless there are extenuating circumstances or provisions to proceed without a Waiver of Confidentiality form, allegations of ethical violations submitted anonymously may or may not be acted upon (ASHA, 2002; AAA, 2003). In general, a complainant should expect that a Waiver of Confidentiality is to be signed because the accused should be provided the opportunity to respond and inform the Board of Ethics that the complaint was not submitted because of malice or ill will (D. R. Denton, personal communication, June 7, 2005).

During Step 6, the board, agency, or employer responsible for investigating the alleged violations must have the cooperation of all interested parties. This process may involve review of records, testimonials, interviews, and other types of fact gathering and documentation. Depending upon the jurisdiction held by the board and/or agency, there could be several types of action taken to resolve the complaint. It is possible for no action to be taken against the professional being accused if there is lack of sufficient evidence or if it is determined that no ethical misconduct has occurred. However, in some cases, sanctions can be serious as in the cases of theft, fraud, or violation of state and federal criminal laws. Is the complaint resolved? Have the desired outcomes been achieved? These questions must be answered by the professional who originally reported the alleged violations. An important part of ethical decision making involves monitoring compliance by the professional found guilty of ethical violations. Who should monitor compliance? How should compliance with imposed sanctions be determined? What if ethical violations continue? What should be done about retaliation, if applicable, against the clinician who reported the ethical violation, that is, the **whistleblower?** If the complaint is not resolved, then it is necessary to review Step 5 and determine which alternative plan of action might be pursued (Step 6 repeated).

All professionals must conduct periodic reviews for changes in the codes of ethics by associations, organizations, or employers. Quality assurance activities and adherence to best practices should reduce the number of ethical violations being observed and reported (Pannbacker, 1998; ASHA Board of Ethics, 2000; ASHA 2005c).

Ethical Dilemmas

Purtilo (1999) described three basic types of ethical problems. First, ethical distress involves facing a challenge about how to maintain one's integrity or the integrity of the profession. Second, an ethical dilemma includes "a challenge about the morally right thing to do; two courses of action diverge" (p. 67). Third, the locus of authority problem involves the challenge faced when deciding who should be the primary decision maker. Case Scenario 4-6 presents an **ethical dilemma.**

CASE SCENARIO 4-6

Mrs. Noble is obtaining therapy services for her four-year-old daughter diagnosed with Down syndrome. Mrs. Noble has her child attending outpatient treatment services two times per week with physical therapy (PT), occupational therapy (OT), and speech-language pathology (SLP) services. A total of six one-hour visits are provided each week. Mrs. Noble asks that the SLP, James, change the dates for treatment on the claims for her daughter's speech-language services for January, February, and

CASE SCENARIO 4-6 *(continued)* ▬▬▬▬▬▬▬▬▬▬▬

March for this year and submit them in April. Mrs. Noble explains that, for claims submitted during the first three months, she will have to pay the deductible and co-pay for those services. Mrs. Noble further explains that she is a single mother of three children and has a job that is very demanding of her time.

Because of layoffs at her work, Mrs. Noble has not received a pay raise for quite some time. She can barely afford to feed the family and pay medical bills. The father of the children does not pay any child support because Mrs. Noble does not know where he is. Mrs. Noble tells James that her daughter is scheduled to have the insertion of pressure equalizing (PE) tubes in February and she wants the deductible to be met with that surgery. Mrs. Noble explains that it will be less out-of-pocket expense for her family if the deductible is met from the surgery because her primary health care company allows only a certain number of visits per year for outpatient therapy services. James asks the mother if she has requested PT and OT to also delay submitting claims for three months. Mrs. Noble says, "I asked the physical therapist last year and she was okay with it, but I don't want to ask her again."

Based on Case Scenario 4-6, what is the ethical distress of the mother and James, the SLP? What is the ethical dilemma of the mother and James? Who should be making the decision about this situation? How would this be explained to James's employer?

The known facts are:

- The child receives treatment from multiple providers.
- The mother asks the SLP to change dates of service to reduce her expense.
- The child is scheduled for surgery.
- The third-party payor covers a limited number of outpatient visits.
- The mother claims that another professional has complied with her request previously.

The questions that are unanswered are:

- What are the details for coverage from the mother's insurance plan?
- Do surgery and treatment services require separate deductibles?
- Did the other professional, in fact, comply with the mother's request?
- What is the child's prognosis?

What are possible ethical violations for James?

- ASHA Principle I: client welfare
- ASHA Principle III: responsibility to the public
- ASHA Principle IV: responsibility to the profession

What are the potential rule violations?

- ASHA Principle I, Rule M: prohibits misrepresentation of services
- ASHA Principle III, Rule D: prohibits misrepresentation and fraud
- ASHA Principle IV, Rule B: prohibits conduct such as dishonesty

What data should James collect/consider?

- Details of the insurance policy
- Relevant codes of ethics/code of business conduct
- Interview with PT
- Functional measure of child's communication

What might the analysis of the data involve?

- Consider the implications of changing dates and potential violations that could involve being reported to the ASHA Board of Ethics and the State Licensure Board.
- Consider alternative actions:
  - Scheduling: Will delaying service delivery for three months impact prognosis?

- Payment: Is an alternative payment schedule possible?
- Help the mother with resources to locate the father so he will pay child support.

What resolutions might be offered?

- Discuss decision to not change dates with mother and ethical violations.
- Provide alternatives to the mother such as postpone treatment until after surgery, modify frequency of visits to fit what the mother can afford, or refer to social/financial services to explore payment options.

Resolution of Ethical Dilemmas

The resolution of ethical dilemmas can be the most difficult step to address in decision making. How do we know which options are best? What suits the case most appropriately? How do we build an argument to justify our choices?

Clinical professionals may utilize the "bioethicist's toolbox," shown in Table 4-1, to reason through and argue about ethical dilemmas (Juengst, 1999). The "tools" include basic arguments of different types and can be used to help a clinician construct convincing positions to discuss and resolve ethical dilemmas. The tools do not presuppose any universal ethical theories directly. Harman (2001) suggests that, rather than choosing a single ethical theory or approach, we must often combine aspects (or tools) in different ways to reason and resolve ethical dilemmas.

Clinicians should recognize that strong arguments and lines of reasoning are used to resolve ethical dilemmas. It is important to understand that total agreement with an opinion, regardless of which "tool" may be used, is not necessary for resolution to occur. Pooser (2002) recommends that clinicians use research, clinical data, and compromise when making ethical decisions and settling disagreements involving family members or clients.

Table 4-1 The Bioethicist's Toolbox

Tool	Ethical Argument/ Statement Used	Example Statement/ Argument
Hammers (driving a decision)	Appeal to shared moral maxims	"Honesty is the best policy."
	Appeal to shared moral principles	"We should promote not harming by avoiding the harms of deception and respect justice for all."
	Appeal to shared traditions	"The professions have a rich history and tradition of helping those with communication disorders."
	Appeal to nonmoral goals	"The foundation of the speech-language-hearing professions is to hold the welfare of the client paramount."
Clamps (bring opinions together)	Arguments from precedent	"Speech-language pathologists try to provide services that are necessary and beneficial."
	Argument by analogy	"Providing additional hearing tests that are not necessary to increase reimbursement is similar to treating a client who will not benefit from services."
	Arguments from clear cases	"Audiologists and speech-language pathologists are taught that intentionally falsifying records in order to justify services is wrong. This is similar to those types of cases."
	Transcendental arguments	"All reasonable people would agree that misinformation and fraud are dishonest and wrong if they had all of the facts."
Wedges (good for prying others away from their opinions)	Exposing consequences	"Providing services that are not necessary and beneficial will undermine the perception that speech-language-hearing professionals are competent and exercise appropriate judgment."
	Exposing implications	"The same type of reasoning could be used to support fraud."

(continued)

Table 4-1 (Continued)

Tool	Ethical Argument/ Statement Used	Example Statement/ Argument
	Exposing inconsistencies	"Bending eligibility guidelines for what is reimbursed by insurance companies could lead to forms of treatment that are not optimal for this particular disorder."
	Exposing biases	"Making a diagnosis is only one role of a speech-language-hearing professional; putting that role first could affect other roles."
Fulcrums (used for pushing a decision in your direction when other opinions have some merit)	Considerations of moral weight	"Confidentiality is very important, but you have to consider whether the client is going to harm someone, and then you have to do what is right."
	Considerations of moral balance	"When considering the total client, it is important to remember that confidentiality can be upheld until the client wants to harm someone else."
	Considerations for moral robustness	"Confidentiality and welfare of the client are paramount, and it is important to consider all aspects and opinions about a client's situation in which he or she threatens to harm someone."
Duct tape (used for patching together a resolution when substantive argument fails)	Negotiating compromises	"Only this one time."
	Appealing to procedure	"How about voting on it?"
	Passing the buck	"Let the boss decide."
Chewing gum (least powerful and persuasive)	Moral introspection	"That's just the way I feel about it."
	Moral hand-wringing	"This is just awful and it is not right."

Reporting Alleged Ethical Violations

Reporting ethical misconduct can take various forms, for example, a face-to-face meeting between two colleagues; reporting the alleged violation to a supervisor; or more formal reporting to an ethics committee, licensure board, or criminal enforcement agency. When the ultimate outcome of reporting an alleged ethical violation is to uphold ethical standards, speech-language-hearing professionals should know why, when, and how to report violations.

Discussion and reporting of an alleged violation could depend upon several factors, such as how to maintain confidentiality of all interested parties, business code of conduct, years of experience a clinician has in the field, rules and procedures established by organizations, and licensing boards, as well as a "level of comfort" that a colleague has with other professionals (Pannbacker, 1998).

ASHA's Council on Professional Ethics (COPE) conducted a survey and concluded that the most common ethical challenges "are the dilemmas of clinical practice and not the behavior of other professionals" (Buie, 1997, p. 3). However, the number of ethical dilemmas occurring in clinical practice and those occurring with other professionals may not reflect the degree of seriousness of an alleged violation. For example, some ethical violations may be resolved between two colleagues with no further discussion involving others. Other situations, however, may be so serious that criminal charges, harm to clients, and loss of public trust are likely to occur.

According to ASHA's Board of Ethics (2000), some alleged ethical violations may be best managed "within individual institutions rather than resorting to local, state, or national reporting or adjudication processes" (p. 93). Reporting alleged ethical violations would provide the framework of an institution a wide range of options to resolve conflicts and develop strategies that may prevent them from reoccurring.

Table 4-2 describes a series of steps that a professional or student may utilize when reporting alleged ethical violations. The steps are not necessarily meant to be on a

Table 4-2 Methods of Reporting Alleged Ethical Violations

Method of Reporting	Example	Issues/Implications
Colleague to colleague	Both colleagues treat same client.	Confidentiality maintained; inexpensive; may have improved communication; potential for retaliation.
Colleague to other team member	Other team member does not treat client but knows client.	Confidentiality compromised; could gain more options from colleague; potential retaliation if colleague talks with others.
Colleague to supervisor	Supervisor knows interested parties.	Confidentiality could be compromised; supervisor informs colleague about rules for reporting and gives options for resolution to colleague.
To institutional ethics committee	Colleague or supervisor (or both) reports alleged violation because previous methods have not resolved issue.	Committee has written procedures for reporting and safeguards against retaliation. Due process procedures can be expensive.
Local, state, or national and adjudication process	Colleague, supervisor, and/or institutional representative may report alleged violation.	Due process procedures are followed; expensive; safeguards against retaliation.

continuum of what is used with less to more serious violations. These steps are recommended as a series of procedures that may result in resolution, be cost-effective, and preserve confidentiality.

Procedures for reporting alleged ethical violations are delineated in formal documents by ASHA (2004) and by the AAA (2003). All professionals and students should review these materials thoroughly prior to submitting a complaint. Similar procedures are usually available from licensing boards and other organizations, such as state speech-language-hearing associations.

The AAA (2003) may require the complainant to "sign a Waiver of Confidentiality that will allow the EPB to disclose his/her name should this become necessary during investigation of the allegation" (p. 4). In certain cases, the EPB of the AAA may act in the absence of a signed Waiver of Confidentiality (e.g., when the EPB has received information that a member is having the license or registration suspended or revoked). ASHA (2004) has similar procedures in that complainant(s) shall submit a signed waiver to the EPB, which allows sending a copy of the complaint to the respondent (the alleged offender) and "consenting to allow to the Board of Ethics to send a copy of the complaint to the Respondent for the Respondent's response" (p. 190). The waiver signed by the complainant allows the EPB of ASHA to send its final decision and any relevant case information to any state agency that licenses or credentials SLPs or AUDs or to any other professional organization "that enforces a Code of Ethics in which the Respondent is a member or applicant for membership" (p. 190). Case Scenario 4-7 presents an alleged ethical violation.

Case Scenario 4-7

As a graduate student in audiology, Donna was asked to submit course evaluations about her professors. All evaluations were done anonymously. Now Donna is employed in a local hospital and is a certified audiologist and a member of ASHA and AAA. She looks for the records of clients who were served by the AUD previously employed by the hospital but cannot locate all of them. The AUD who worked at the hospital has moved to another state. When Donna contacted the AUD, she was told, "I couldn't keep up with all of the paperwork. My focus was upon the clients improving. Some of the clients' folders have enough information." Donna is angry about the lack of record keeping and decides that this is a serious ethical violation and writes a letter to the ethics boards of ASHA and AAA but does not sign her letter. Because her return address is on the outside of the envelope, she receives letters from ASHA's and AAA's ethics boards requesting that she sign a Waiver of Confidentiality. Donna does not feel she should sign it because when she did evaluations about course instructors, she did not have to provide her name.

Why should Donna sign the waiver? What are her options if it is not signed? What other resolutions may be contemplated? What information from the "bioethicist's toolbox" may be used to resolve this dilemma?

Before addressing these questions, one should review the facts that are known:

- Donna is a member of ASHA and of AAA and is bound by their codes of ethics.
- Donna cannot locate all of the records for clients seen by an AUD who was previously employed by the hospital.
- The previously employed AUD admits that some records are incomplete.
- Donna reports to ASHA and AAA about poor record keeping of the other AUD and does not sign the letter, thinking it should be anonymous.
- Donna receives requests to sign a Waiver of Confidentiality from ASHA and AAA in order to continue their investigations.

What questions are unanswered at this time?

- Is the AUD who was employed previously by the hospital a member of ASHA and/or AAA?
- Has Donna sought any legal counsel about signing the form?

Why should Donna sign the waiver?

- Because Donna is bound to the codes of ethics, she is obligated to uphold responsibilities to the profession (ASHA Principle I) and dignity of the profession (AAA Principle 8). ASHA Principle IV, Rule J (comply with the Board of Ethics), and AAA Rule 8d (cooperate with the Ethical Board) also factor into Donna's decision to sign the Waiver of Confidentiality form.
- Donna signs the form because she is concerned about ASHA Principle 1 (welfare of clients) and AAA Principle 3 (maintain confidentiality and adequate records).

What if Donna decides not to sign the Waiver of Confidentiality form?

- Donna could be reprimanded by ASHA and AAA ethics boards for not cooperating because she has already filed a written complaint.

- Donna does not sign the form, and ASHA and AAA cease to investigate the case any further. Dignity of the profession is compromised, and the AUD previously employed by the hospital is not held accountable for these actions.

What other resolutions may be contemplated?

- Donna contacts the AUD and explains to her the importance of upholding ethics and that she should work on improving this in her practice.

- Donna sends a letter to the employer of the AUD and states that this person had difficulty maintaining adequate records. She does sign the letter.

What information from the "bioethicist's toolbox" may be used to address this dilemma?

- Hammers: Donna tries to "drive a decision" by the other AUD and convinces her that, as a profession, they should hold the welfare of the client paramount. Donna convinces the AUD that it would be best if they worked together to reconstruct the client information that is missing in the files.

- Wedges: Donna tries "prying others away from their opinions" and states to the other AUD that she will expose the poor record keeping. The other AUD agrees that she will help reconstruct the records to avoid being reported to ASHA and AAA.

- Chewing gum: Donna states that "this is not right" and decides not to sign the Waiver of Confidentiality form, and the investigation does not proceed.

There are a variety of "tools" that may be used in ethical dilemmas. Generally, it is best to convince all interested parties by using the strongest "tools" (hammers, wedges).

Individual responsibility should be paramount in choosing which "tools" are utilized and in letting ethical principles and rules guide one's choices.

Ethics Enforcement

ASHA, AAA, licensing boards, state speech-language-hearing associations, employers, and other organizations with written codes of ethics and/or codes of conduct have a variety of options that can be taken after a careful review of all information. These options are listed in Table 4-3 and Table 4-4.

Sanctions vary in severity. Relatively modest infractions may involve an educative letter, censure, or a letter of reprimand. The harshest penalties by ASHA are revoking membership and/or certification. The most significant penalty by AAA and state speech-language-hearing associations is revoking membership. State licensing boards can impose a variety of sanctions, including revoking of licensure and reporting certain cases to criminal enforcement agencies and/or third-party payors. Businesses and other work settings can impose a variety of sanctions for ethical violations that have been proven, including dismissal from job duties. The jurisdiction of one board, agency, or organization is not necessarily bound by all of the same codes of ethics or laws; therefore, individual cases may be treated and resolved differently (ASHA, 2002; Denton, 2002).

Monitoring compliance by anyone found guilty of ethical violations is an ongoing process. The responsibility of who shall do the monitoring is not always clear. In cases in which discussion occurred only between two colleagues and went no farther, there should be mutual respect that any corrections to clinical practice will be maintained by the violator. In cases in which supervisors; ethics committees at work; or state, local, or national boards are involved, the process should fall to the entity that rendered the decision.

Appeals to the entity with the jurisdiction to enact any penalty are always an option. ASHA (2004) describes

Table 4-3 Possible Outcomes and Sanctions for Ethical Violations Enforced by ASHA (2002)

Outcome	Definition
Case review	Evidence for ethical violation is not sufficient and case is closed. Respondent and complainant are informed.
Initial determination	Initial determination by the Board of Ethics, subject to further consideration and appeal, of the (1) finding, (2) proposed action, and (3) extent of disclosure.
Sanctions imposed	Reprimand; censure; withhold, suspend, or revoke membership and/or Certificate of Clinical Competence; or other measure determined by the Board of Ethics at its discretion. A cease and desist order may become part of any action.
Disclosure	Upon becoming final, the Board of Ethics decision shall be published in an ASHA publication, distributed to all membership, and shall be provided to any person or entity requesting a copy, if the sanction is censure, or the withholding, suspension, or revocation of membership and/or Certificate(s) of Clinical Competence. For reprimand, the decision is disclosed only to respondent, respondent's counsel, complainant(s), witnesses at the Board of Ethics further consideration hearing, staff, and association counsel.
Further consideration	Respondent may request that the Board of Ethics give further consideration to the initial determination.
Board of Ethics decision	Final decision of the Board of Ethics after (1) further consideration or (2) thirty days from the date of notice of the initial determination by the Board of Ethics if no request for further consideration is received.
Appeal	Written request from respondent to the Board of Ethics alleging error in the Board of Ethics decision and asking that it be reversed in whole or in part by the Executive Board.
Reinstatement	Person whose membership or certification has been revoked may apply for reinstatement at the completion of the revocation period.

Table 4-4 Possible Outcomes and Sanctions for Ethical Violations Enforced by AAA (2003)

Outcome	Definition
Insufficient evidence	Ethical Practice Board (EPB) determines there is insufficient evidence of an ethical violation, the parties are notified, and the case is closed.
Sanctions	Educative letter, cease and desist order, reprimand, mandatory continuing education, probation of suspension, suspension of membership, revocation of membership (after one year may reapply for membership but not guaranteed).
Appeal	Member may appeal final finding and decision of the EPB to the AAA Board of Directors with its decision being final.
Education of membership	Upon majority vote, the EPB can decide to have circumstances and nature of cases presented in *Audiology Today* and in the Professional Resource area of the AAA Web site (http://www.audiology.org). The member's identity will not be made public.

an appeals process that can be used by its members and/or certificate holders. Other cases may involve the court system and include numerous parties and other agencies.

Summary

Ethical decision making is usually a complicated process that a clinician probably faces several times during a career. It is important that the decisions being made follow a logical process that guides the clinician in collecting relevant information, considering several plans of action, determining which plan is best to use, and implementing and evaluating the plan. Reporting an ethical dilemma should not be done in haste or with malice. It is important that each decision be carefully considered and that it make use of available resources.

References

American Academy of Audiology. (2003). *Code of ethics of the American Academy of Audiology.* Retrieved from http://www.audiology.org.

American Speech-Language-Hearing Association. (2002). Ethical practice inquiries: ASHA jurisdictions. *ASHA Supplement, 22.*

American Speech-Language-Hearing Association. (2004). *Statement of practices and procedures of the Board of Ethics.* Retrieved from http://www.asha.org.

American Speech-Language-Hearing Association. (2005a). *Background information and standards and implementation for the Certificate of Clinical Competence in speech-language pathology.* Retrieved from http://www.asha.org.

American Speech-Language-Hearing Association. (2005b). *New audiology standards.* Retrieved from http://www.asha.org.

American Speech-Language-Hearing Association. (2005c). *Quality indicators for professional service programs in audiology and speech-language pathology [Quality Indicators].* Retrieved from http://www.asha.org.

American Speech-Language-Hearing Association Board of Ethics. (2000). In response to "Whistleblowing in speech-language pathology by M. Pannbacker." *American Journal of Speech-Language Pathology, 9,* 93–94.

Buie, J. (1997). Clinical ethics survey shows members grapple with ethical dilemmas. *ASHA Leader,* 3.

Chabon, S. S., & Morris, J. F. (2004, February 17). A consensus model for making ethical decisions in a less-than-ideal world. *ASHA Leader,* 18–19.

Denton, D. R. (2002, May 28). How to file an ethics complaint. *ASHA Leader.* Retrieved from http://www.asha.org.

Denton, D. R. (personal communication, June 7, 2005).

Gabard, D. L., & Martin, M. W. (2003). *Physical therapy ethics.* Philadelphia: F. A. Davis.

Harman, L. B. (2001). *Ethical challenges in the management of health information.* Gaithersburg, MD: Aspen.

Juengst, E. (1999). The bioethicist's toolbox. *Centerviews: The Newsletter of the Center for Bioethics at Case Western Reserve University, 10,* 5–6. Retrieved from http://www.cwru.edu.

Kilmas, N. (2001, November). Ethical issues span practice settings: From telemedicine to academia. *Advance for Speech-Language Pathologists and Audiologists,* 7–8, 19.

Pannbacker, M. (1998).Whistleblowing in speech-language pathology. *American Journal of Speech-Language Pathology,* 7(4), 18–23.

Pannbacker, M., & Irwin, D. L. (2003, July). *Ethics for speech-language pathologists and audiologists.* Teleseminar presented by the American Speech-Language-Hearing Association.

Pooser, P. B. (2002, November 19). When clinician and parent disagree. *ASHA Leader.* Retrieved from http://www.asha.org.

Purtilo, R. (1999). *Ethical dimensions in the health professions.* Philadelphia: W. B. Saunders.

Weinstein, B. (2001, November). Thinking through questions of ethics: Four steps to better decision making. *Advance for Speech-Language Pathologists and Audiologists,* 28–29.

Chapter 5

Beneficence
and
Nonmaleficence

Learning Objectives
After reading this chapter, you should be able to:

- Understand and apply ethical principles related to beneficence and nonmaleficence.
- Analyze related case studies.
- Make appropriate clinical decisions.

Introduction

Beneficence means doing good or being kind. The principle of beneficence means that professionals should always try to help clients and protect them from harm (do no harm, nonmaleficence). Speech-language pathologists (SLPs) and audiologists (AUDs) seek to benefit those persons they serve professionally and take care to do no harm. These persons include clients, research participants, colleagues, students, supervisors, and other professionals. Speech-language pathologists and audiologists seek to safeguard the welfare and rights of those persons they serve professionally. When ethical issues or problems occur, SLPs and AUDs are responsible for taking reasonable steps to resolve issues and problems. Both the AAA (2003) and ASHA (2003) codes of ethics have principles and rules related to beneficence and nonmaleficence. These principles and rules are presented in Table 5-1.

Table 5-1 **Principles and Rules Related to Beneficence and Nonmaleficence from the AAA (2003) Code of Ethics and the ASHA (2003) Code of Ethics**

AAA	Operational Description	ASHA
2	Competence	I-A
2b	Referral	I-B
1b	Avoiding discrimination	I-C
1, 6a, 7a	Fidelity, honesty	I-D
2d	Delegation of duties	I-E
5	Full disclosure	I-F
5b	Effectiveness of services, and products	I-G
5b	Avoiding guarantees	I-H
—	Correspondence	I-I
—	Telecommunication	I-J
5e	Documentation	I-K
3	Confidentiality	I-L
4b	No charge for services not rendered	I-M
4d	Informed consent	I-N
—	Substance abuse	I-O

This chapter covers a number of case scenarios related to doing good and avoiding harm. The following sections provide an extensive selection of case studies that illustrate many of the principles and rules of either the Code of Ethics of ASHA or of the AAA.

General focus questions need to be asked in order to make decisions about cases. This includes answers to the following questions:

1. What information is needed to identify and scrutinize the problem?
2. What are the possible courses of action?
3. Is there a need for consultation? If so, what type of consultation?
4. How will the plan of action be implemented and monitored?

These questions are based on the model of ethical decision making described in Chapter 4. In addition, specific information on a case-by-case basis is needed. Each of the case scenarios has guidelines and suggestions to consider.

Several of the scenarios include Vee diagrams (Gowin & Alvarez, 2005; Novak, 1998). A Vee diagram provides a framework for organizing information and for analyzing and resolving problems. These case analyses may serve as useful references in making ethical decisions about the hypothetical cases as well as in professional practice.

Welfare of Persons Served

Both the ASHA and AAA codes of ethics give highest consideration to the welfare of persons served professionally. This ethical principle is first in order of appearance and in order of guidance for ethical decision making. The fundamental question for SLPs and AUDs is, "Who are the persons I serve professionally?" (Helmick, 2000, p. 46).

SCENARIO 5-1 ▬▬▬▬▬▬▬

A speech-language pathologist (SLP) is doing a research project with children. The SLP administers some language tests and then asks the children to give a description of something that they would like to see different at home. (See Figure 5-1.)

Points to Consider

1. What if the child reveals something that is very sensitive in nature?
2. Is it appropriate to ask this question?
3. What ethical standards are involved?

Suggestions

1. Review the ASHA (2003) Code of Ethics, especially Principle I, Rule L.

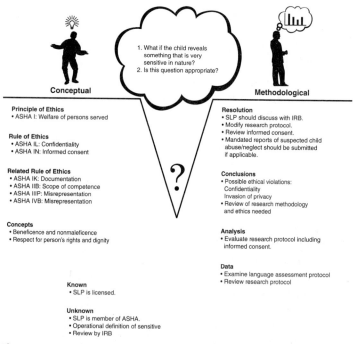

Figure 5-1 Vee diagram for welfare of persons served: speech-language pathology. (Scenario 5-1)

2. Be aware of informed consent issues (Antoine, 2002).
3. Review ASHA's issues in ethics statements: "Ethics in Research and Professional Practice" (2002a) and "Protection of Human Subjects" (2005b).

SCENARIO 5-2

An audiologist has been in practice for twenty-five years and continues to perform all diagnostic testing as he learned it in school. (See Figure 5-2.)

Points to Consider

1. Have audiology procedures changed in the past twenty-five years?
2. Could clients be harmed by using older procedures?

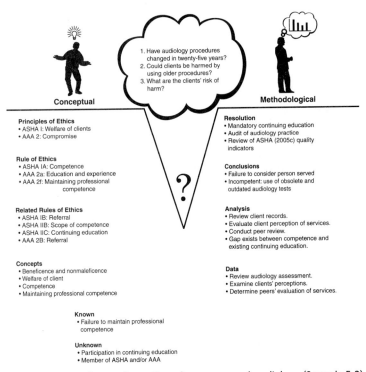

Figure 5-2 Vee diagram for welfare of persons served: audiology. (Scenario 5-2)

3. What are the clients' risks of harm?
4. Could this situation have an impact on certification? Licensure? Accreditation?
5. Who is responsible for resolving this situation?

Suggestions

1. Review codes of ethics, especially standards related to maintaining competence and continuing education.
2. Review AAA and ASHA position statements, guidelines, and technical reports.
3. Develop and implement a plan for maintaining competence (Golper & Brown, 2004).
4. Find a mentor to advise and monitor continuing education.

Competence

Standards of competence are based on the ethical principles of beneficence and nonmaleficence. Competence is the ability to provide a level of care according to a standard of care and according to the profession's code of ethics (Aiken, 2002).

SCENARIO 5-3

An SLP earned a master's degree and the CCC about fifteen years ago, and an adult with a swallowing disorder is referred. During the master's degree program, this SLP did not receive any instruction about swallowing disorders. (See Figure 5-3.)

Points to Consider

1. Should the SLP provide services to this client?
2. What are the appropriate options for this SLP?
3. Does the SLP have post-graduate training and experience in dysphagia?

Suggestions

1. Consult the ASHA Web site about dysphagia practice and issues.

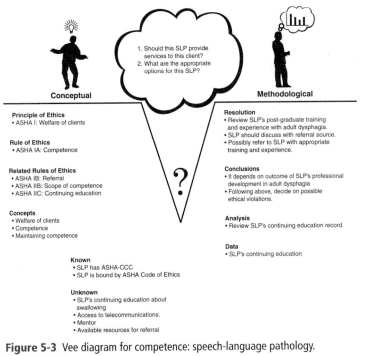

Figure 5-3 Vee diagram for competence: speech-language pathology. (Scenario 5-3)

2. Review ASHA's (2002b) "Knowledge and Skills Needed by Speech-Language Pathologists Providing Services to Individuals with Swallowing and/or Feeding Disorders."

3. Consider topics for graduate curriculum for pediatric and adult dysphagia identified by ASHA's (1997a) Special Interest Division: "... Swallowing and Swallowing Disorders."

4. Read *Dysphagia,* the professional journal dedicated to swallowing and swallowing disorders.

SCENARIO 5-4

An AUD has heard about a new hearing aid and believes that it will help a client. Use of this hearing aid requires specialized fitting procedures that the AUD has not learned.

Points to Consider

1. Can the AUD provide services competently?
2. Is it in the best interest of the client to be fitted with the latest technology?
3. How could this dilemma be resolved?

Suggestions

1. Review and apply information about evaluating diagnostic and treatment procedures (ASHA, 2005c), as well as relevant in-service materials from the manufacturer.
2. Consult recent peer-reviewed research about the hearing aid.
3. Refer to an AUD who is qualified with the hearing aid by training and experience.
4. Consult AAA's Code of Ethics, especially Principle 1, Rule 2a and Rule 2b.
5. Consult ASHA's Code of Ethics, especially Principle I, Rules A, B, F, and G.

Consultations and Referrals

Speech-language pathologists and audiologists should use every available resource including referrals to ensure high-quality service. The current codes of ethics of ASHA (2003) and AAA (2005) contain specific reference to referral: Rule I-B and Rule 2b, respectively.

SCENARIO 5-5

A mother reports during a diagnostic interview that there is a family history of bipolar disorder.

Points to Consider

1. What should the SLP do?
2. Who would be the appropriate referral source?

Suggestions

1. Obtain further information: such as relevance to client's problem.

2. Review ASHA's (2001b) *Scope of Practice in Speech-Language Pathology.*
3. Consult ASHA's (2003) Code of Ethics, especially Rule I-B.
4. Consider referral for multidisciplinary evaluation or referral to medical source to assess appropriateness of psychiatry referral.

SCENARIO 5-6

An AUD has been working for six months with an infant who has a hearing impairment. Every time the mother brings the baby to see the AUD, she weeps uncontrollably and laments the "life" her child is facing. The AUD refers her to a grief counselor and a parent support group.

Points to Consider

1. Does this seem necessary?
2. Could the AUD provide the necessary counseling?

Suggestions

1. Consult AAA's (2003) Code of Ethics, especially Rule 2b.
2. Consult ASHA's (2003) Code of Ethics, especially Rule I-B.
3. Provide parent education materials.
4. Review ASHA (1997b) *Preferred Practice Patterns for Audiology.*
5. Review ASHA's (2004c) *Guidelines for the Audiologic Assessment of Children from Birth to 5 Years of Age.*
6. Consult reference materials about counseling, such as Kendall (2000), Luterman (2001), McNamara (2002), and Shames (2000).

Discrimination

Discrimination is showing prejudice or partiality in the delivery of professional services. Speech-language pathologists and audiologists should not deny persons service based on factors such as gender, race or ethnicity, religion, national origin, sexual orientation, or disability. Discrimination is specifically addressed by ASHA's (2003) Code of Ethics through Rule I-B and AAA's (2005) Code of Ethics through Rule 1b.

SCENARIO 5-7

A client is referred to the clinic because of a possible voice disorder. The male client reveals that he is transgendered and would prefer to speak with a higher-pitched voice. The SLP states that there may be other clinicians who can help. This could be unfair discrimination based on sexual orientation. On the other hand, it could be that the SLP does not have appropriate training/experience in treatment of voice problems. (See Figure 5-4.)

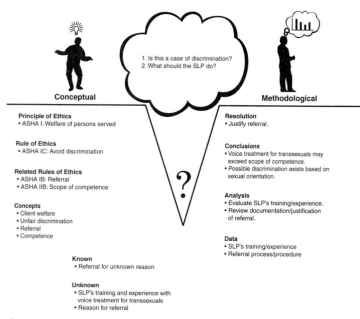

Figure 5-4 Vee diagram for discrimination: speech-language pathology. (Scenario 5-7)

Points to Consider

1. Is this a case of discrimination?
2. Does the SLP have the requisite training and experience?
3. What should the SLP do?

Suggestions

1. Review ASHA Code of Ethics (2003), especially Rule I-C.
2. Read relevant information about the voice of transsexual individuals in Boone and McFarlane (2000) and Case (2002).

SCENARIO 5-8

An AUD does not believe that she can competently deliver services to an individual who only speaks Spanish. (See Figure 5-5.)

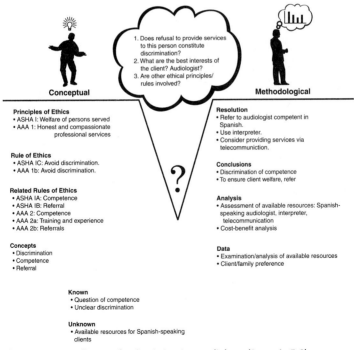

Figure 5-5 Vee diagram for discrimination: audiology. (Scenario 5-8)

Points to Consider

1. Does refusal to provide services to this person constitute discrimination?
2. What are the best interests of the client? The AUD?
3. Are there ethical principles/rules involved?

Suggestions

1. Develop reference list of common terms in Spanish.
2. Consult with university foreign language department.
3. Seek help from interpreter.
4. Enroll in Spanish conversational course.

Accuracy of Credentials

Speech-language pathologists and audiologists are responsible for providing accurate information about both their own credentials and those of assistants, technicians, and support personnel.

SCENARIO 5-9

An SLP with a CCC has employed a speech-language pathology assistant.

Points to Consider

1. What kind of identification should the assistant wear?
2. How should reports be signed?
3. What credentials should be used by the SLP assistant?
4. What should be done if the state licensure board provides no guidelines about informing the public about employment of an SLP assistant?

Suggestions

1. Consult ASHA's Code of Ethics, especially Rule I-D.
2. Review the state licensure board's regulations for assistants and support personnel.
3. Review ASHA's (2004i) statement on support personnel.

SCENARIO 5-10 ▬▬▬▬▬▬▬▬▬▬▬▬▬▬▬▬▬▬▬▬▬

Two summer interns were working with an AUD, primarily doing observations. As the summer progressed, they began helping clients complete case history forms. They wore name badges identifying their status and introduced themselves as student interns when they met clients. The client was told that the AUD would review the case history and conduct the test.

Points to Consider

1. Were the interns appropriately identified?
2. Who was responsible for reviewing and interpreting the case history?
3. Did the AUD interview the client about his or her history?

Suggestions

1. Review ASHA and AAA codes of ethics, I-D and I-E, and 2a, respectively.
2. Ensure that the AUD is responsible for obtaining and interpreting the client's case history.

Delegation of Work to Others

Speech-language pathologists and audiologists who delegate work to assistants, technicians, support personnel, or students take steps to (1) avoid delegating tasks requiring professional competence and (2) see that the services are adequately supervised.

SCENARIO 5-11 ▬▬▬▬▬▬▬▬▬▬▬▬▬▬▬▬▬▬

An SLP, living in a remote rural area of the United States with a large caseload, has employed a part-time employee with a degree in speech communication. This is permitted by the state licensure board, but the SLP wants to have the employee do speech-language screenings for a local school system.

Points to Consider

1. What should the SLP do to avoid any ethical violations?
2. How much supervision should be provided?
3. Where would the SLP go for guidelines and rules?

Suggestions

1. Review the ASHA Code of Ethics, especially I-E and I-J.
2. Consider telepractice. See ASHA's (2004g, 2004h, 2005a) statement and report on telepractice.

SCENARIO 5-12

Consider the previous audiology case study (Scenario 5-10).

Points to Consider

1. Is the task assigned to the summer interns appropriate for their skill level?
2. How do you know?
3. Are they adequately supervised?
4. Should a client's first contact be with a support person or with a professional?

Suggestions

1. Review procedures and competencies for obtaining case history information.
2. Document and verify skill level and supervision.
3. Ensure that interns are familiar with procedures for maintaining client confidentiality.
4. Follow HIPAA guidelines.
5. Review relevant principles and rules from ASHA and AAA codes of ethics, such as I-E, I-J, and I-L; and 2d, and 3, respectively.

Full Disclosure

Speech-language pathologists and audiologists should provide persons with information about the nature and possible effects of services or products and participation in research.

SCENARIO 5-13

An SLP is conducting a research project with adolescents who have a diagnosis of autism spectrum disorder and language delay.

Points to Consider

1. What is (are) the procedure(s) for informing these adolescents about the possible effects of the research?
2. Should other people be consulted to provide consent? Who would they be?

Suggestions

1. Follow IRB protocol, including informed consent.
2. Consult ASHA (2002a), "Ethics in Research and Professional Practice."
3. Consult ASHA's (2003) Code of Ethics, especially I-N.

SCENARIO 5-14

The hearing aid that an AUD is going to use with a client is capable of producing enough gain to damage hearing. The hearing aid was programmed at a level that would not cause damage.

Points to Consider

1. Does the AUD need to inform the client that the hearing aid is capable of causing damage?
2. Will the hearing aid hurt the client at the adjusted settings?

Suggestions

1. Consult AAA's Code of Ethics, especially Rule 2c.
2. Consult ASHA's Code of Ethics, especially Rule I-F.
3. Develop a plan to monitor hearing aid status.

Effectiveness of Services and Products

Effectiveness of services and products can be determined by cost-benefit analysis. This is an evaluation comparing the cost of service or products with the benefits. Effective treatment has been described as: the problem is completely eliminated, the severity of the problem is reduced, or the problem is stable but the client has learned an alternative but effective means of communicating (Lum, 2002).

Scenario 5-15

A child with very poor speech intelligibility is being served by an SLP. The SLP is meeting with the mother and making the recommendation for an augmentative communication system. The electronic speech-generating device being considered would be used both at home and school.

Points to Consider

1. What should the SLP do to address the mother's concerns that the device will benefit her child?
2. What should the SLP do about evaluating the effectiveness of the service?

Suggestions

1. Consult ASHA's (2003) Code of Ethics, especially Rule I-G.
2. Review *Preferred Practice Patterns* for augmentative and alternative communication (ASHA, 2004d) and roles and responsibilities of SLPs with respect to augmentative and alternative communication (ASHA, 2001a, 2004f).

Scenario 5-16

An AUD uses programming software which graphically displays anticipated improvement in hearing for the client.

Points to Consider

1. Is this sufficient to evaluate the effectiveness of the hearing aid?

2. What other ways can the AUD use to evaluate the effectiveness of this product?

Suggestions

1. Consult AAA's (2003) Code of Ethics, especially Principle 4 and Principle 5.
2. Consult ASHA's (2003) Code of Ethics, especially I-G.
3. Review AAA's (2004) "Guidelines for Ethical Practice in Research for Audiologists," especially the section on product-oriented outcomes research.
4. Assess client perceptions, i.e., quality of life.

Avoiding Guarantees

Speech-language pathologists and audiologists must avoid guarantees that are false, misleading statements about their services, products, or research findings.

SCENARIO 5-17

An SLP works for a rehabilitation services company and is very excited about the treatment program developed by a supervisor that has helped many adults with verbal apraxia of speech. The SLP informs the client that this program has been successful with many people and will help him speak more clearly.

Points to Consider

1. How could the SLP evaluate the effectiveness of this treatment program?
2. Do you think that the SLP has committed an ethical violation?
3. If so, what should be done to correct it?

Suggestions

1. Review the ASHA (2003) Code of Ethics, especially I-H, III-B, and III-D.
2. Has information about this program been published in peer-reviewed journals?
3. What type and level of evidence are available?
4. Review ASHA's (2004a) *Evidence-Based Practice in Communication Disorders*.

Scenario 5-18

When a new hearing aid becomes available, an AUD uses an Internet training site prepared by the manufacturer to learn how to fit the hearing aid and its benefits. The manufacturer proclaims that this hearing aid is effective in managing background noise. When the AUD tells a client about the hearing aid, he indicates that the hearing aid has been found effective in background noise.

Points to Consider

1. Does this constitute an implied guarantee of the results?
2. Is this only a reasonable statement of prognosis?
3. What criteria could you use to make a distinction?

Suggestions

1. Review the AAA (2003) Code of Ethics, especially Principle 2 and Principle 4, and Rule 4e and Rule 5b.
2. Review the ASHA (2003) Code of Ethics, especially I-H, III-B, and III-D.
3. Search peer-reviewed journals for information about benefits of this hearing aid.
4. Consider type and level of evidence.
5. Consult ASHA's (2004a) introduction to evidence-based practice.

Avoid Providing Services Solely by Correspondence

Speech-language pathologists and audiologists do not provide services solely by correspondence.

Scenario 5-19

A friend of an ASHA-certified SLP calls and asks several questions about speech-language treatment for a nephew who has a history of otitis media. The friend thanks the SLP for the information and then hangs up.

Points to Consider

1. What should the SLP do?
2. Have any ethical violations occurred?
3. If so, describe.

Suggestions

1. Review the ASHA (2003) Code of Ethics, especially I-B and I-I.
2. The SLP should discuss and document the need to refer for medical evaluation and treatment.

SCENARIO 5-20

A man from Florida told a friend about purchasing hearing aids from an AUD in Arkansas. The friend contacted this AUD about obtaining an audiogram and ear mold impressions by a local AUD and then ordering his hearing aids by mail as he had learned that the cost of a similar hearing aid in Florida would be much higher.

Points to Consider

1. What should the Arkansas AUD say?
2. Why might hearing aids be more expensive in one location than in another?
3. What service issues are problematic with "long-distance" fittings that may explain the need for the rule of ethics regarding not providing services solely by correspondence?

Suggestions

1. Review AAA (2003) Code of Ethics, especially Principle 4 and Principle 5 and Rule 5a.
2. Consider ASHA (2003) Code of Ethics, especially Rule I-B and Rule I-I.
3. Be aware of responsibility for hearing aid fitting and repair.

Telecommunication

Telepractice is the use of technology to provide professional services at a distance (ASHA, 2005a). Prerequisites for telepractice are knowledge and skills about telepractice models, technology associated with service delivery, matching clients to technology, selecting assessments and treatments appropriate to the technology, cultural/linguistic variables, use of support personnel, evaluation of service effectiveness, and documentation of services.

SCENARIO 5-21

An SLP has established a Web page that provides general information about speech and language disorders. The Web page has information about developmental milestones and indicators about potential delays. An e-mail address is provided for people to contact the SLP with questions.

Points to Consider

1. Under what conditions may this situation be an ethical violation?
2. What should the SLP do about HIPAA regulations? See Chapter 3 for a brief discussion of HIPAA or see http://www.hhs.gov for extensive information about national standards to protect the privacy of personal health information.

Suggestions

1. Obtain clarification of response to questions.
2. Determine relation of answers to clinical services.
3. Review ASHA (2003) Code of Ethics relative to telecommunication, Rule I-J.
4. Review ASHA (2004g, 2004h, 2005a) reports about telepractice.
5. Consult state licensure standards about telepractice because it is prohibited by some state boards.

SCENARIO 5-22

Mr. Jones received his hearing aid from Mr. Smith, an AUD, when he lived in his town. He subsequently moved thirty miles away, and it is difficult for him to come in for appointments. Mr. Smith and Mr. Jones talked on the phone about adjustment problems he was having. After three phone calls, Mr. Smith recommended that Mr. Jones come in for additional programming of his hearing aid. The state that they live in does not prohibit practice by telephone.

Point to Consider

1. Is there any problem with providing service in this manner?

Suggestions

1. Inventory available equipment and resources.
2. Review ASHA's (2004g, 2004h, 2005a) guidelines related to telecommunication.
3. Consider AAA (2003) Code of Ethics which does not directly mention telecommunication although there are several related guidelines relevant to competence, training, and experience.

Documentation

The importance of documentation in speech-language pathology and audiology cannot be overemphasized. Documentation is required for all professional activities including clinical services, research, supervision, and continuing education.

SCENARIO 5-23

A school-based SLP maintains records in a locked file cabinet. A supervisor with the State Department of Education comes and states that she must review folders to evaluate adequacy of record keeping. The state department representative shows official identification to verify her position. The SLP allows her to review the records of ten students.

Points to Consider

1. What ethical violations may have occurred?
2. What are some other things the school-based SLP should have done in this situation besides ask for identification?

Suggestions

1. Consult ASHA's (2003) Code of Ethics, especially Rule I-K and Rule I-L.
2. Review school policy and procedures for documenting access to records.

SCENARIO 5-24

An AUD has been seeing a child whose parents are divorcing. The child's father has been bringing the child for evaluation and treatment services for the last six weeks. His mother recently requested a copy of the records.

Points to Consider

1. Is she entitled to the records?
2. How can you determine if she is authorized?

Suggestions

1. Review ASHA (2003) Code of Ethics, especially Rule I-K and Rule I-L.
2. Review AAA (2003) Code of Ethics, especially Principle 3, Rule 3a.
3. Consult legal services.

Confidentiality

Confidentiality extends to all professional activities: teaching, service, and research. **Breach of confidentiality** occurs when someone who has legitimate access to information shares it with others who have no legitimate reason to know (Aiken, 2002). However, information can be released without consent if mandated by law or governmental regulations. Speech-language pathologists and audiologists should know about confidentiality requirements of HIPAA (Golper & Brown, 2004).

SCENARIO 5-25

A forty-six-year-old male is referred for voice treatment to a community-based SLP. During a treatment session, the patient discloses that he has suicidal thoughts because he is unhappy about his life.

Points to Consider

1. What should the SLP do?
2. Under what conditions might this information be shared with others?
3. Should other professionals be consulted or would that be an ethical violation?

Suggestions

1. Encourage the client to consult his family physician.
2. Refer the client (with his consent) for psychological-psychiatric services.
3. Consult legal services trained to handle referrals for clients with mental health concerns, who are mentally disturbed.
4. Maintain an ethical balance between safeguarding client welfare and right to privacy.
5. Review ASHA's (2003) Code of Ethics relative to benefiting those with whom we work and taking care to do no harm: Principle I, Rule I-B, Rule I-L.

SCENARIO 5-26

Two AUDs are visiting in a social situation. Both have seen the same client but at different times, and they share information about the client.

Points to Consider

1. Since they have both seen the client, is it alright to share information?
2. Under what conditions could this be permissible?
3. Does the environment change the nature of their exchange in any way?
4. Could it be possible for others to overhear their exchange?
5. Would that be a violation of confidentiality?

Suggestions

1. Avoid exchanging confidential information in nonprofessional contexts because nonprofessional situations increase risk of breach of confidentiality.
2. Recognize the breach of confidentiality if client did not authorize release of information.

3. Review ASHA (2003) and AAA (2005) codes of ethics; both consider confidentiality: I-L and 3, 3a, respectively.

Fees for Services

Speech-language pathologists and audiologists cannot charge for services not provided, products not dispensed, or research activities not conducted. As early as possible in a clinical or research relationship, SLPs, AUDs, and recipients of these services should reach an agreement about compensation and billing. ASHA has provided related guidelines about clinical services provided by students and clinical fellows and obtaining insurance reimbursement or funding (ASHA, 2004b, 2004c, 2004i). AAA also has several guidelines and advisories relative to fees that are available on their Web site at http://www.audiology.org.

SCENARIO 5-27

An SLP has just begun the clinical fellowship (CF) and is informed by his supervisor that he can bill for services while planning for client services provided in a nursing home (including while driving to the facility).

Point to Consider

1. What should the SLP say to the supervisor?

Suggestions

1. Review ASHA (2003) Code of Ethics, Rule I-M.
2. Document request.
3. Inform supervisor of violation of Code of Ethics (Rule I-M); this would be violation of Rule IV-A: "... prohibit anyone under their supervision from engaging in any practice that violates the Code of Ethics" (p. 15).
4. Report ethical misconduct to licensure board and ASHA.

SCENARIO 5-28

A speech and hearing clinic at a university charges for treatment services on a semester basis. The client pays one fee ($200) at the beginning of the semester for fifteen treatment sessions. The client misses six sessions during the semester.

Points to Consider

1. Is it an ethical violation to charge for services not rendered?
2. What should be done?
3. How might this be handled by the supervisor or student?

Suggestions

1. Review ASHA (2003) Code of Ethics, Rule I-M.
2. Provide financial management in accordance with established policies and procedures.
3. Provide documentation of providing financial policies/procedures to client.

SCENARIO 5-29

An AUD uses a test that is considered controversial. ASHA has indicated that use of the procedure is permissible as part of a research study of efficacy.

Point to Consider

1. Should clients sign an informed consent for permission to participate in a research project?

Suggestions

1. Consult AAA's (2003) Code of Ethics, especially Rule 4a and Rule 4d.
2. Accurately inform client of services rendered. See ASHA (2003) Code of Ethics, Rule I-M.
3. Document informed consent and the experimental nature of test.
4. Reduce or do not charge for experimental services.

Informed Consent

Informed consent is a legal and ethical duty to provide information about clinical services and research in an understandable fashion to clients. The minimum standards of what constitutes informed consent can be found in the ethical codes of AAA (2003) and ASHA (2003).

Informed consent reflects respect for client **autonomy.** Information (disclosure) requirements include: nature, purpose and type of procedure(s) to be used; risks and benefits; alternatives to treatment; consequences of no treatment; financial cost(s); and any additional information the client may request (Aiken, 2002; Gabard & Martin, 2003).

SCENARIO 5-30

An SLP videotaped a treatment session with a child to demonstrate a treatment program to graduate students in speech-language pathology.

Points to Consider

1. What should be done?
2. Would consent be required if the SLP also interviewed the parents?

Suggestions

1. Review Rule I-N of the ASHA (2003) Code of Ethics.
2. Obtain informed consent for teaching demonstration.

SCENARIO 5-31

After collecting clinical data, an AUD decides that the results have merit in evaluating the outcome of clinical services and can be analyzed and submitted for publication in a professional journal.

Points to Consider

1. Should this AUD inform subjects that their data will be used in a research project?
2. Is it acceptable to obtain consent after data are collected?
3. Is there ever a reason for exempting data from this restriction?

Suggestions

1. Review AAA's (2003) Code of Ethics, Rule 2 and Principle 3, and "Guidelines for Ethical Practice in Research for Audiologists" (AAA, 2004).
2. Review ASHA (2003) Code of Ethics, Rule I-N.
3. Consult Institutional Review Board.
4. Be aware of informed consent issues in research (Antoine, 2002; Meline, 2006).

Substance Abuse

Speech-language pathologists and audiologists should refrain from professional activities when they know or should know that there is likelihood that substance abuse or other health-related conditions will adversely affect their professional activities.

SCENARIO 5-32

A clinician who holds the CCC-SLP is employed by a private clinic. Co-workers and adult clients have repeatedly noticed that the clinician has slurred speech, stumbling gait, and visual perceptual problems.

Points to Consider

1. What types of conditions may produce symptoms similar to those described?
2. Is the clinician aware of these problems?
3. Is the clinician receiving treatment for these problems?

Suggestions

1. Defer action until relevant information about the problem is available.
2. Consider facility guidelines as well as HIPAA and ADA.

SCENARIO 5-33

The senior audiologist where you are employed has a long history of alcohol abuse including several DWIs. There are acute episodes which are frequently obvious during professional activities.

Points to Consider

1. What steps have been taken by the audiologist about this problem? What steps have been taken by the employer?
2. What should be done by other employees if the employer chooses not to intervene?

Suggestions

1. Review facility policy as well as other guidelines such as ASHA, AAA, HIPAA, and ADA.
2. Contact AA about strategies for co-workers of persons who are alcohol dependent.
3. Consider other professional opportunities.

Summary

Case studies/scenarios related to beneficence and nonmaleficence were presented in this chapter and covered such topics as competence, referral, discrimination, delegating duties, prognosis, avoiding guarantees, correspondence, telecommunication, informed consent, and substance abuse. Some ethical dilemmas are obvious, and others are less obvious and require careful consideration and possibly consultation. Furthermore, most case studies are multidimensional, that is, they involve multiple ethical principles and rules.

Identifying ethical issues and dilemmas of hypothetical cases can improve ethical decision making as well as resolution of ethical dilemmas. Case studies can be analyzed by individual SLPs and AUDs or by groups for analysis and comparison.

References

Aiken, T. D. (2002). *Legal and ethical issues in health occupations*. Philadelphia: W. B. Saunders.

American Academy of Audiology (2003). Code of ethics and procedures, rules and penalties. Retrieved May 19, 2006, from, http://www.audiology.org.

American Academy of Audiology. (2004). Guidelines for ethical practice in research for audiologists. *Audiology Today, 15*(6), 14–17.

American Speech-Language-Hearing Association. (1997). Graduate curriculum on swallowing and swallowing disorders (adult and pediatric dysphagia). *ASHA Desk Reference, 3*, 348a–348n.

American Speech-Language-Hearing Association (1997b). Preferred practice patterns for the profession of audiology. Retrieved May 26, 2006, from http://www.asha.org.

American Speech-Language-Hearing Association. (2001a). Augmentative and alternative communication: Knowledge and skills for service delivery. *ASHA Supplement, 22*, 97–106.

American Speech-Language-Hearing Association. (2001b). *Scope of practice in speech-language pathology*. Rockville, MD: Author.

American Speech-Language-Hearing Association. (2002a). Ethics in research and professional practice. *ASHA Supplement, 22*, 63–64.

American Speech-Language-Hearing Association. (2002b). Knowledge and skills needed by speech-language pathologists providing services to individuals with swallowing and/or feeding disorders. *ASHA Supplement, 22*, 81–88.

American Speech-Language-Hearing Association. (2003). Code of ethics. *ASHA Supplement, 23*, 13–15.

American Speech-Language-Hearing Association. (2004a). *Evidence-based practice in communication disorders*. Retrieved May 19, 2006, from http://www.asha.org.

American Speech-Language-Hearing Association. (2004b). Fees for clinical service provided by students and clinical fellows. *ASHA Supplement, 24*, 49–50.

American Speech-Language-Hearing Association. (2004c). *Guidelines for the audiologic assessment of children from birth to 5 years of age*. Retrieved May 19, 2006, from http://www.asha.org.

American Speech-Language-Hearing Association. (2004d). *Preferred practice patterns for the profession of speech-language pathology*. Retrieved May 19, 2006, from http://www.asha.org.

American Speech-Language-Hearing Association. (2004e). Representation of services for insurance reimbursement or funding. *ASHA Supplement, 24*, 51–53.

American Speech-Language-Hearing Association. (2004f). *Roles and responsibilities of speech-language pathologists with respect to augmentative and alternative communication: Position statement*. Retrieved May 19, 2006, from http://www.asha.org.

American Speech-Language-Hearing Association. (2004g). *Speech-language pathologists providing clinical services via telepractice: Position paper.* Retrieved May 19, 2006, from http://www.asha.org.

American Speech-Language-Hearing Association. (2004h). *Speech-language pathologists providing clinical services via telepractice: Technical report.* Retrieved May 19, 2006, from http://www.asha.org.

American Speech-Language-Hearing Association. (2004i). *Support personnel.* Retrieved May 19, 2006, from http://www.asha.org.

American Speech-Language-Hearing Association. (2005a). *Knowledge and skills needed by speech-language pathologists providing clinical services via telepractice.* Retrieved May 19, 2006, from http://www.asha.org.

American Speech-Language-Hearing Association. (2005b). *Protection of human subjects (Issues in ethics).* Retrieved May 19, 2006, from http://www.asha.org.

American Speech-Language-Hearing Association. (2005c). *When evaluating any treatment procedure, product, or program.* Retrieved May 19, 2006, from http://www.asha.org.

Antoine, M. P. (2002). Informed consent issues. In T. D. Aiken (Ed.), *Legal and ethical issues in health occupations* (pp. 57–74). Philadelphia: W. B. Saunders.

Boone, D. R., & McFarlane, S. C. (2000). *The voice and voice therapy.* Needham Heights, MA: Allyn & Bacon.

Case, J. L. (2002). *Clinical management of voice disorders.* Austin, TX: Pro-Ed.

Gabard, D. L., & Martin, M. W. (2003). *Physical therapy ethics.* Philadelphia: F. A. Davis Company.

Golper, L. A., & Brown, J. E. (2004). *Business matters: A guide for speech-language pathologists.* Rockville, MD: American Speech-Language-Hearing Association.

Gowin, D. B., & Alvarez, M. C. (2005). *The art of educating with V diagrams.* Cambridge: Cambridge University Press.

Helmick, J. W. (2000). Professional ethics and audiology. In H. Hosford-Dunn, R. J. Rosser & M. Valente (Eds.), *Audiology practice management* (pp. 41–48). New York: Thieme.

Kendall, D. L. (2000). Counseling in communication disorders. *Contemporary Issues in Communication Science and Disorders, 27,* 96–103.

Lum, C. (2002). *Scientific thinking in speech and language therapy.* Mahwah, NJ: Lawrence Erlbaum Associates.

Luterman, D. M. (2001). *Counseling persons with communication disorders and their families.* Austin, TX: Pro-Ed.

McNamara, K. M. (2002). Interviewing, counseling, and clinical communication. In R. Paul (Ed.), *Introduction to clinical methods in communication disorders* (pp. 183–217). Baltimore: Brookes Publisher.

Meline, T. (2006). *Research in communication sciences and disorders.* Upper Saddle River, NJ: Pearson Education.

Novak, J. D. (1998). *Learning, creating, and using knowledge: Concept Maps as Facilitative Tools in Schools and Corporation.* Mahwah, NJ: Lawrence Erlbaum Associates.

Shames, G. H. (2000). *Counseling the communicatively disabled and their families: A manual for clinicians.* Boston: Allyn & Bacon.

Chapter 6

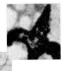

Competence

Learning Objectives

After reading this chapter, you should be able to:

- Understand and identify issues related to professional competence.
- Make ethical decisions about standard of care.

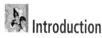 Introduction

Competence is the ability to provide a level of care according to a standard of care and according to the professional's code of ethics (Aiken, 2002). The standards of competence are based on the ethical principles of beneficence (do good) and nonmaleficence (avoid harm) (Knapp & Vande-Creek, 2006).

The second Principle of Ethics in ASHA's (2003) Code of Ethics involves competence and has six supporting statements (see Table 6-1). These standards essentially require speech-language pathologists (SLPs) and audiologists (AUDs) to achieve and maintain the highest level of professional competence. In the AAA (2003) Code of Ethics, there are also standards dealing with competence (also shown in Table 6-1): Lack of competence could result in disciplinary action from ASHA's Board of Ethics, the AAA, a state speech and hearing association, or a state licensure board; SLPs and AUDs only provide services, teach, and conduct research in areas within their scope of competence based on their education, training, and experience; no SLP or AUD is competent in all areas of practice (ASHA, 2001a, 2004e). Speech-language pathologists and audiologists benefit from discussions about scope of practice and scope of competence from time to time.

Golper and Brown (2004) suggest that SLPs and AUDs maintain a written list of competencies that identify areas

Table 6-1 Principles and Rules Related to Competence from the 2003 AAA Code of Ethics and the 2003 ASHA Code of Ethics

AAA	Operational Description	ASHA
2	Competence	II
	Certification	II-A
2a	Education and experience	II-B
2c	Continuing education	II-C
2d	Supervision and delegation	II-D
		II-E
—	Maintenance of equipment	II-F

of practice in which they are competent to provide services, teach, and conduct research. Such a list can be useful in verifying necessary qualifications for specific areas of practice in SLP or AUD.

Highest Level of Professional Competence

Speech-language pathologists and audiologists are responsible for achieving and maintaining the highest level of professional competence. Competence to teach, provide clinical services, and conduct research may be gained through education, training, or supervised experience.

SCENARIO 6-1

An SLP who is a clinical researcher is unaware of the 2003 revision of ASHA's Code of Ethics.

Points to Consider

1. What areas of professional practice are at risk for ethical misconduct?
2. How could—and why should—this situation be resolved?

Suggestions

1. Review ASHA's (2003) Code of Ethics.
2. Consult ASHA's (2004b) *Guidelines for Verifying Competencies in Speech-Language Pathology.*
3. Review "The Ethics of Competence" (Mustain, 2003).

SCENARIO 6-2

An AUD never looks at the revisions of the Code of Ethics or Practice Guidelines developed by ASHA.

Points to Consider

1. Is this AUD maintaining the highest level of professional competency?
2. What if the AUD is adhering to AAA's standards?

3. Are there differences between AAA and ASHA standards?
4. Should an AUD consider the standards of both organizations?
5. What if the AUD only belongs to one of these associations?

Suggestions

1. Review the codes of ethics (AAA, 2003; ASHA, 2003).
2. Develop a strategic plan for updating ethical knowledge and associated skills (Golper & Brown, 2004).

Certificate of Clinical Competence

Speech-language pathologists and audiologists can engage in the provision of clinical services only when they hold the appropriate Certificate of Clinical Competence (CCC) or when they are in the certification process and are supervised by an individual who holds the appropriate CCC.

Scenario 6-3

An SLP is asked by the employer to conduct hearing screenings for children seen at the clinic. The SLP is also asked to interpret an audiogram sent to the school by the health unit. The SLP interprets the audiogram.

Points to Consider

1. What ethical violations occurred?
2. How could this be prevented ?

Suggestions

1. Review ASHA's (2001a) *Scope of Practice in Speech-Language Pathology.*
2. Consult ASHA's (2003) Code of Ethics, especially Principle II, Rule A.
3. Clarify the nature of the conflict; make known your commitment to ASHA's Code of Ethics.

4. Consider balancing ethical responsibilities and employee demands (ASHA, 2003).
5. Review "Employers, Employees and Ethics" in the October 7, 2003, *ASHA Leader.*
6. Review ASHA's (2004a) Issues in Ethics statement: "Clinical Practice by Certificate Holders in the Profession in Which They Are Not Certified."

Scenario 6-4

ASHA has begun the process of requiring continuing education to maintain the Certificate of Clinical Competence (CCC).

Points to Consider

1. If an individual does not earn the necessary continuing education units (CEUs), is his or her CCC still valid?
2. Will hours that the individual supervises count for practicum credit?
3. Is this AUD adhering to required professional standards?
4. What if this AUD lives in a remote area and is unable to attend CEU events?
5. Is there a hardship exclusion?
6. Should there be? Why or why not?
7. Does ASHA-approval-of-CEUs imply endorsement of content? When might this be problematic?

Suggestion

1. Review ASHA and AAA documents such as practice statements and certificate standards, which are available on both organizations' Web sites.

Scope of Competence

Speech-language pathologists and audiologists should engage in only those aspects of the professions that are within the scope (boundaries) of their competence, considering their level of education, training, and experience.

SCENARIO 6-5 ▬▬▬▬▬▬▬▬▬▬▬▬▬▬

An SLP is working for a rehabilitation agency that serves several skilled nursing facilities. The SLP is referred patients with Alzheimer's disease but has not received any formal training about the disease and related communication disorders.

Points to Consider

1. What should be done in the short term and in the long term?
2. Should telecommunication be considered?

Suggestions

1. Review ASHA (2003) Code of Ethics, especially Principle I, Rule A (competence), Rule B (referral), and Rule J (telecommunication).
2. Provide mentorship with an experienced/trained SLP.
3. Review ASHA (2001b, 2004f) reports about providing services through telecommunication.

SCENARIO 6-6 ▬▬▬▬▬▬▬▬▬▬▬▬▬▬

The recent move to universal infant hearing screening in the newborn nursery means that there is an increasing number of babies coming to AUDs at a very early age for hearing aid fittings.

Points to Consider

1. Should an AUD who is comfortable fitting children who are two or three years old fit children who are much younger?
2. What if no other AUDs in the area are experienced in fitting very young children?
3. How could expertise be developed?

Suggestions

1. Obtain competence-based continuing education.
2. Read literature relevant to universal hearing screening, such as that which is available on ASHA and AAA Web sites.

Continuing Education

Speech-language pathologists and audiologists are expected to continue their professional development throughout their careers. In other words, SLPs and AUDs are expected to embrace lifelong learning and will often need to develop skills beyond those developed during graduate education or during the clinical fellowship (Mustain, 2003). There are several options for continuing education in speech-language pathology and audiology: workshops, in-service presentations, college/university courses, consultation with other SLPs and AUDs, attending professional meetings, reading professional journals and books, utilizing Internet resources, viewing videotapes and listening to audiotapes, using tutorial software, and doing clinical outcome research (Silverman, 2003).

SCENARIO 6-7

An SLP has been providing services for several years to children who use augmentative communication devices. It has been several years since the SLP has attended any training about new devices that are on the market.

Points to Consider

1. What should be done by the SLP?
2. What ethical violations may arise besides continuing professional development?

Suggestions

1. Know the roles and responsibilities of SLPs related to augmentative/alternative communication (AAC) (ASHA, 2004d).
2. Consider continuing education options.
3. Participate in mentorship with an SLP knowledgeable about AAC.

SCENARIO 6-8

ASHA currently requires continuing education to maintain the Certificate of Clinical Competence in audiology.

Audiologists who received the ASHA CCC prior to 1980 were required to participate in thirty contact hours of professional development activities in the three-year period from January 1, 2003, to December 31, 2005.

Points to Consider

1. How can CEUs be documented?
2. What happens if the AUD does not earn the required CEUs?
3. What are the requirements for reinstating the ASHA CCC?

Suggestion

1. Review ASHA's continuing education requirements for maintaining certification.

Delegating Duties

Speech-language pathologists and audiologists delegate the provision of clinical services only to: (1) persons who hold the appropriate CCC; (2) persons in the education or certification process who are appropriately supervised by an individual who holds the appropriate CCC; or (3) assistants, technicians, or support personnel who are adequately supervised by an individual who holds the appropriate CCC.

SCENARIO 6-9

An SLP is the owner of a local rehabilitation company. Several years ago, the SLP let the CCC lapse. The SLP has employed two SLP-CFY clinicians and does not disclose that her certification is not current with ASHA. At the end of the CF, the clinicians are told by ASHA that their supervisor is not currently certified.

Points to Consider

1. What should be done?
2. Who is responsible for taking action?
3. Who would be consulted?

Suggestions

1. Review ASHA/CCC requirements that specify that CFs are responsible for verifying CCC status of CF supervisor.
2. Know how to file an ethics complaint (Denton, 2002).
3. Report violations to ASHA's Board of Ethics and the state licensure board.

SCENARIO 6-10

An individual misrepresents herself as holding the CCC in audiology, and a recent graduate takes a job with her for supervision of the clinical fellowship year. At the end of the year, when forms are submitted, the graduate learns that her experience will not count.

Points to Consider

1. Does the graduate have any recourse for completing her clinical fellowship year?
2. How can an individual determine the status of a professional's CCC?
3. How might one assess whether there is legal liability?
4. Is this an issue for a licensure board?
5. Is this an issue for ASHA's Board of Ethics?

Suggestion

1. Consider suggestions in Scenario 6-9.

Scope of Competence

Speech-language pathologists and audiologists shall not require or permit their professional staff to provide services or conduct research activities that exceed the staff members' competence, level of education, training, and experience.

SCENARIO 6-11

Treating patients with a tracheotomy is required as part of a job in a local hospital. This information was made known during an interview. An SLP working with children for several years decides to accept this job. After two weeks, the supervisor of the new employee requires a patient with a tracheotomy to be seen in the ICU.

Points to Consider

1. What should the new employee do?
2. How would the ethical dilemma be resolved for the supervisor and the supervisee?

Suggestions

1. Take reasonable steps to move into this new area of practice.
2. Explain to employees the consequences of ethical violations such as practicing outside one's professional scope of competence.
3. Provide the employee with appropriate options to provide this service, including continuing education, consultation, and/or telecommunication.
4. Review how employees can balance ethical responsibilities and employer demands (Huffman, 2003).
5. Consider ASHA's (2005) quality indicators for clinical service program.

SCENARIO 6-12

A recent graduate in audiology is assigned by his employer to a nursing home for hearing screening, hearing aid maintenance, and aural rehabilitation services. Several residents at the nursing home have swallowing problems, and the company tells the AUD to provide services so that another professional will not need to be assigned to that facility.

Points to Consider

1. What can the AUD do?
2. Could refusal jeopardize employment?
3. Is there a good way to handle the problem?

Suggestion

1. Explain to the employer the consequences of clinical practice in a profession in which one does not hold certification (ASHA, 2004a).

Maintenance of Equipment

Speech-language pathologists and audiologists ensure that all equipment used in the provision of services or to conduct research and scholarly activities is in proper working order and is properly calibrated. In other words, SLPs and AUDs do not use out-of-order or uncalibrated equipment in teaching, service, or research.

SCENARIO **6-13**

An SLP in a community-based center provides hearing screenings but, due to budgetary problems, has not had the portable audiometer calibrated in two years. The supervisor of the SLP does not support having the audiometer calibrated because of continuing budget problems.

Points to Consider

1. What should the SLP do about this situation?
2. What if the supervisor requires the SLP to do hearing screenings for another few months and thinks there will be money to have it calibrated?

Suggestions

1. Explain to the supervisor that using an uncalibrated audiometer would be an ethical violation. Also note that, for clients with speech-language problems, failure to screen hearing or refer for audiology evaluation is a violation and not considered good clinical practice.
2. Review ASHA's (2004c) *Preferred Practice Patterns for the Profession of Speech-Language Pathology.*
3. Borrow or rent an audiometer.

Scenario 6-14

After employment, an AUD requests copies of equipment calibration records and learns that the equipment has not been properly checked for two years.

Points to Consider

1. Are the tests done valid?
2. What can be done about previous evaluations?
3. Can the tests be considered valid if calibration indicates the equipment is performing within specifications?

Suggestions

1. Review ASHA's (1997, 2005) *Preferred Practice Patterns for the Profession of Audiology* and quality indicators for clinical service programs.
2. Recall and retest all clients tested during this two-year period.

Summary

The major focus of this chapter was professional competence in speech-language pathology and audiology. Related case studies/scenarios were presented: maintaining competence, Certificate of Clinical Competence, continuing education, delegating duties, scope of competence, and maintaining equipment. For each case study, points to consider and suggestions were provided.

References

Aiken, T. D. (2002). *Legal and ethical issues in health occupations.* Philadelphia: W. B. Saunders.

American Academy of Audiology. (2003). *Code of ethics and procedures, rules, and penalties.* Retrieved May 19, 2006, from http://www.audiology/org.

American Speech-Language-Hearing Association. (1997) *Preferred practice patterns for the profession of audiology.* Rockville, MD: Author.

American Speech-Language-Hearing Association. (2001a). *Scope of practice in speech-language pathology.* Rockville, MD: Author.

American Speech-Language-Hearing Association. (2001b). *Telepractice and ASHA: Report of the telepractice team.* Rockville, MD: Author.

American Speech-Language-Hearing Association. (2003). Code of ethics. *ASHA Supplement, 23,* 13–15.

American Speech-Language-Hearing Association. (2004a). Clinical practice by certificate holders in the profession in which they are not certified. *ASHA Supplement, 24,* 39–40.

American Speech-Language-Hearing Association. (2004b). *Guidelines for verifying competencies in speech-language pathology.* Rockville, MD: Author.

American Speech-Language-Hearing Association. (2004c). *Preferred practice patterns for the profession of speech-language pathology.* Retrieved May 19, 2006, from http://www.asha.org.

American Speech-Language-Hearing Association. (2004d). Roles and responsibilities of speech-language pathologists with respect to augmentative and alternative communication. *ASHA Supplement, 24,* 93–95.

American Speech-Language-Hearing Association. (2004e). Scope of practice in audiology. *ASHA Supplement, 24,* 27–35.

American Speech-Language-Hearing Association. (2004f). *Speech-language pathologists providing clinical services via telepractice: Technical report.* Retrieved May 19, 2006, from http://www.asha.org.

American Speech-Language-Hearing Association. (2005). *Quality indicators for professional programs in audiology and speech-language pathology.* Retrieved May 19, 2006, from http://www.asha.org.

Denton, D. R. (2002, May 28). How to file an ethics complaint. *ASHA Leader.* Retrieved May 23, 2006, from http://www.asha.org.ethics.

Golper, L. A., & Brown, J. E. (2004). *Business matters: A guide for speech-language pathologists.* Rockville, MD: American Speech-Language-Hearing Association.

Huffman, N. P. (2003, October 7). *Employers, employees, and ethics.* ASHA Leader. Retrieved May 23, 2006, from http://www.asha.org.ethics.

Knapp, S. J., & VandeCreek, L. D. (2006). *Practical ethics for psychologists*. Washington, DC: American Psychological Association.

Mustain, W. (2003, June 24). The ethics of competence. *ASHA Leader, 8*, 12.

Silverman, F. H. (2003). *Essentials of professional issues in speech-language pathology and audiology*. Prospect Heights, IL: Waveland Press.

Chapter 7

Public Statements

Learning Objectives

After reading this chapter, you should be able to:

- Discuss standards of ethical conduct related to public statements.
- Identify ethical issues in public statements.
- Apply ethical decision making to public statements.

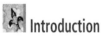 Introduction

Speech-language pathologists (SLPs) and audiologists (AUDs) have an obligation to the public and other professionals to provide accurate and relevant information about any aspect of the professions. They do not misrepresent their credentials, competence, education, training, experience, or scholarly and research contributions. They are alert to and guard against potential conflicts of interest.

Furthermore, public announcements and statements such as advertising, announcements, and marketing of professional services should provide accurate and adequate information to aid the public in making informed choices about speech-language pathology and audiology service (ASHA, 2003). SLPs and AUDs should not make false or misleading statements to the public or other professionals. The ASHA (2003) and AAA (2003) codes of ethics provide guidance concerning these issues. SLPs and AUDs should make professional judgments in the best interests of those they serve, such as clients, students, research participants, supervisees, and other professionals. A comparison of these principles and rules is shown in Table 7-1. The ethical dilemmas in this chapter are related to public statements and include misrepresentation, conflicts of interest, and promotional activities.

Table 7-1 Principles and Rules Related to Public Statements/ Communication for AAA (2003) and ASHA Codes of Ethics (2003)

AAA	Operational Definition	ASHA
6	Communication	III
6a	Accurate information:	III-A
7a	Credential, competency, training, experience, scholarly research contributions	
4c	Conflict of professional interest	III-B
6b	Financial conflicts of interest	III-C
	Avoid misrepresentation	III-D
	Accurate public statements	III-E
6b	Advertisements, announcements, marketing	III-F

General focus questions need to be asked in order to make decisions about cases. These include the following questions:

1. What information is needed to identify and scrutinize the problem?
2. What are the possible courses of action?
3. Is there a need for consultation? If so, what type of consultation?
4. How will the plan of action be implemented and monitored?

Representation of Credentials

It is important in building trust from the public that speech-language-hearing professionals be truthful about their credentials, competence, education, training, experience, and scholarly or research contributions. Public trust could be quickly compromised if members and the public discovered that ASHA-certified and AAA members are not totally honest either in written or oral communication.

SCENARIO 7-1

An SLP has a job as director of a speech and hearing department in a large hospital. The SLP lists credentials including the CCC in SLP and AUD. The SLP holds the CCC-SLP; however, the SLP only holds a license as a hearing aid dispenser in another state and does not hold the CCC-AUD.

Points to Consider

1. What should be done?
2. How might this be resolved?

Suggestions

1. Review the paper regarding clinical practice by certificate holders in the profession in which they are not certified (ASHA, 2004a).

2. Review *Scope of Practice in Speech-Language Pathology* (ASHA, 2001) and *Scope of Practice in Audiology* (ASHA, 2004f).
3. Review *Public Announcements and Public Statements* (ASHA, 2002e).
4. Review the state licensing law and discuss the scope of practice (National Council of State Board of Examiners for Speech Language Pathology and Audiology [NCSB], 2006).

SCENARIO 7-2

An AUD falsely advertises that he has received specialty certification in cochlear implants through the American Academy of Audiology. Although he has attended several continuing education workshops on cochlear implants, he has not taken the required test administered by AAA for this certification.

Points to Consider

1. Is he misrepresenting his credentials?
2. What reprimand might he receive?

Suggestions

1. Review the Code of Ethics (AAA, 2003) and the procedures for management of alleged violations.
2. Review the book *Ethics in Audiology: Guidelines for Ethical Conduct in Clinical, Educational, and Research Settings* (AAA, 2003).

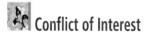 Conflict of Interest

Speech-language pathologists and audiologists should take caution not to engage in professional activities that constitute a conflict of interest. The professional needs to be sensitive to the fact that perceptions of a conflict of interest may be viewed negatively by the public. The **code of conduct** for employees may also have specific rules regarding conflicts of interest.

SCENARIO 7-3 ▬▬▬▬▬▬▬▬▬▬▬▬▬▬▬▬▬

An SLP is employed full time as a clinical supervisor at a university. The SLP also is in a group private practice in the same town. A mother says that she needs to have her child seen for treatment as soon as possible and the clinic at the university does not have any available slots. The SLP refers the mother to the private practice group but does not have the case assigned to her.

Points to Consider

1. Is this an ethical violation?
2. What else should be done?

Suggestions

1. Review *Drawing Cases for Private Practice from Primary Place of Employment* (ASHA, 2002b).
2. Review *Quality Indicators for Professional Service Programs in Audiology and Speech-Language Pathology* (ASHA, 2005c).
3. Consult the state licensing board rules and regulations regarding drawing cases for private practice from primary place of employment (NCSB, 2006).
4. Review *Conflicts of Professional Interest* (ASHA, 2004c).
5. Review the code of conduct for employees of the university.

SCENARIO 7-4 ▬▬▬▬▬▬▬▬▬▬▬▬▬▬▬▬▬

An AUD with a CCC-AUD and a member of AAA is offered an all-expense-paid trip to the Bahamas by a hearing aid company for the purpose of training in fitting new hearing aids.

Points to Consider

1. Will accepting this offer obligate the AUD to fit these aids?
2. Does this give the appearance of a conflict of interest?
3. What might clients think if they knew about this trip?

Suggestions

1. Review the papers from AAA including the advisories regarding buying groups, rewards, trips, cash rebates, and conflicts of interest (AAA, 2004a, 2004b); ethical practice guidelines on financial incentives from hearing instrument manufacturers (AAA, 2004c); and the book *Ethics in Audiology: Guidelines for Ethical Conduct in Clinical, Educational, and Research Settings* (AAA, 2006).
2. Review the paper, *Conflicts of Professional Interest* (ASHA, 2004c).
3. Review the rules and regulations from the state licensing board regarding conflicts of professional interest (NCSB, 2006).

Financial Conflict of Interest

It is important for SLPs and AUDs to understand that clients should be served professionally solely on the basis of those being referred and not on any financial interest of the professional. Financial interest may include actual currency or goods and services.

SCENARIO 7-5

An adult with aphasia has been referred to a local outpatient clinic. The outpatient clinic offers an array of therapy services including physical therapy, occupational therapy, and speech-language treatment. The client is informed that there are several other clinics available in the same town for services, but many do not have an SLP with extensive experience. The SLP talks with the family and provides a list of workshops he has attended in the last five years about aphasia.

Points to Consider

1. Is this an ethical dilemma?
2. If yes, what problems do you see with the situation?
3. What might the client or the client's family think about the comments made about the other outpatient clinics?

Suggestions

1. Review the papers *Public Announcements and Public Statements* (ASHA, 2002e) and *Conflicts of Professional Interest* (ASHA, 2004c).
2. Review and discuss *Model Bill of Rights for People Receiving Audiology or Speech-Language Pathology Services* (ASHA, 1993); *Knowledge and Skills Needed by Speech-Language Pathologists Providing Services to Individuals with Cognitive Communication Disorders* (ASHA, 2005a); and *Definition of ASHA's Continuing Education Unit* (ASHA, 2002a).

SCENARIO 7-6

An AUD participating in a citywide health fair chooses to refer only those people who have the potential for purchasing a high-priced digital hearing aid to his private practice for further testing. All others are referred to a state-supported institution.

Points to Consider

1. Is it in the best interest of lower income clients to receive services that are state supported?
2. How could the AUD handle this situation in an unbiased manner?

Suggestions

1. Review and discuss the papers *Competition* (ASHA, 2004b) and *Rights and Responsibilities of Test Takers: Guidelines and Expectations* (ASHA, 2002f).
2. Review the book *Ethics in Audiology: Guidelines for Ethical Conduct in Clinical, Educational, and Research Settings* (AAA, 2005).

Reporting Professional Information

Professional information is related to diagnosis, research, services rendered, or products dispensed. Also, it is important that there be no plans to defraud in connection with obtaining reimbursement. Products sold or services rendered by an SLP or an AUD shall not be obtained illegally.

Scenario 7-7 ▬▬▬▬▬▬▬▬▬▬▬▬▬▬▬▬▬▬▬▬

An SLP with a CCC and a membership in the state speech-language-hearing association provides services in a private practice and offers a 20 percent discount for payments made in cash. When the SLP bills the third party for reimbursement, the total fee is charged (not including the discount).

Points to Consider

1. Should this be done?
2. Does this practice of billing constitute an ethical violation? If so, what type of crime is committed?
3. Might this practice have legal implications?

Suggestions

1. Review and discuss the papers *Competition* (ASHA, 2004b); *Conflicts of Professional Interest* (ASHA, 2004c); and *Representation of Services for Insurance Reimbursement or Funding* (ASHA, 2004e).
2. Review the state speech-language-hearing association's code of ethics for its membership and the licensing law for the state (NCSB, 2006).

Scenario 7-8 ▬▬▬▬▬▬▬▬▬▬▬▬▬▬▬▬▬▬▬▬

A client's insurance company reimburses the cost of hearing aids and professional services if the hearing loss was due to an accident at the client's place of employment. The client's AUD, who holds the CCC-AUD and is a member of AAA, indicates that the cause of the hearing loss was work related to ensure payment of these services, but she does not have adequate documentation.

Points to Consider

1. How could work-related hearing loss be documented?
2. Is the AUD jeopardizing the relationship with the insurer?
3. Are there obligations to the insurer? To the insured?

Suggestions

1. Review and discuss the papers *Guidelines on the Audiologist's Role in Occupational and Environmental Hearing Conservation* (ASHA, 1996); *Business, Marketing, Ethics, and Professionalism in Audiology: An Updated Annotated Bibliography* (1986–1989) (ASHA, 1991); and *Representation of Services for Insurance Reimbursement or Funding* (ASHA, 2004e).
2. Review the book *Ethics in Audiology: Guidelines for Ethical Conduct in Clinical, Educational, and Research Settings* (AAA, 2005).

Description of Services

It is imperative that SLPs and AUDs provide the public accurate information. This includes any information that is disseminated regarding the nature and management of communication disorders, the professions, professional services, research, and scholarly activities. Public trust is developed when the information is complete and unbiased.

SCENARIO 7-9

A university faculty member with the CCC-SLP is conducting a research study and is advertising for participants in the local newspaper. The announcement does not include the information that all participants will disclose previous sexual history.

Points to Consider

1. What are the ethical violations that may occur?
2. How could the advertisement have been changed?

Suggestions

1. Review and discuss the papers *Protection of Human Subjects* (ASHA, 2005b); *Ethics in Research and Professional Practice* (ASHA, 2002c); and *Rights and Responsibilities of Test Takers: Guidelines and Expectations* (ASHA, 2002f).
2. Submit all advertisements to the Institutional Review Board (IRB) for approval prior to dissemination.

SCENARIO 7-10

Mr. Williams has just received the AuD, doctorate of audiology, degree through a distance learning program. In an informational lecture to a group of senior citizens at a hospital seminar on good health, Mr. Williams boasts that an audiologist with an AuD can diagnose specific vestibular disorders in patients without the consultation of an ENT physician because of advanced diagnostic tools that audiologists use on a daily basis.

Points to Consider

1. Can an AUD do what Mr. Williams claims to do?
2. How would a client that is treated without an ENT and is dissatisfied with the services make it known?

Suggestions

1. Review the book *Ethics in Audiology: Guidelines for Ethical Conduct in Clinical, Educational, and Research Settings* (AAA, 2006).
2. Review *Scope of Practice in Audiology* (ASHA, 2004f) and *Public Announcements and Public Statements* (ASHA, 2002e).

Standards of Reporting

The use of announcements, and marketing to the public by SLPs and AUDs shall adhere to the prevailing professional standards. The "prevailing standard" is not specifically described by the codes of ethics for ASHA and AAA. Information about professional services, reporting research results, and promoting products must not include any misrepresentations so the public can make informed choices.

SCENARIO 7-11

In the *Yellow Pages*, a licensed SLP states: "state-certified swallowing therapist"; however, the licensure board does not provide specific endorsement or specialty recognition.

Points to Consider

1. What should be done by the SLP, other SLP professionals, and the state licensure board?
2. How might the public react if they learn that this type of an endorsement does not exist?

Suggestions

1. Review the papers *Public Announcements and Public Statements* (ASHA, 2002e) and *Ethics in Research and Professional Practice* (ASHA, 2002c) and state licensing laws rules and regulations (NCSB, 2006).
2. Review and discuss the paper *Knowledge and Skills Needed by Speech-Language Pathologists Providing Services to Individuals with Swallowing and/or Feeding Disorders* (ASHA, 2002d).
3. Discuss what should be done when ASHA offers specialty recognition for swallowing and feeding but a state licensure board does not offer such recognition.

SCENARIO 7-12

An AUD collecting data for a research project on hybrid cochlear implants reports that her method of programming the speech processor is producing incredible results. She also states that the results surpass other implants, even though the data do not fully support this conclusion.

Points to Consider

1. Is it ethical for this AUD to report conclusive findings on partial data?
2. How might the results be re-stated?

Suggestions

1. Review and discuss *Ethics in Research and Professional Practice* (ASHA, 2002c); *Technical Report: Cochlear Implants* (ASHA, 2004h); and *Public Announcements and Public Statements* (ASHA, 2002e).
2. Review the book *Ethics in Audiology: Guidelines for Ethical Conduct in Clinical, Educational, and Research Settings* (AAA, 2006).

3. Review the technical report regarding the use of evidence-based practice in communication disorders (ASHA, 2004d).

Summary

Public trust for the professions of speech-language pathology and audiology is gained and secured by the actions of all professionals in the fields. Professional organizations, licensure boards, and the code of conduct for employees of various employment settings hold the importance of truth to the public in very high regard. It is possible that public trust can be compromised by criminal actions, poor professional judgments, and/or lack of telling the truth. Consultation with colleagues about truth in advertisements and/or public statements can help ensure that the perception by the public is held with regard to the prevailing standards.

Some of the issues discussed in this chapter may seem relatively clear in determining how an ethical dilemma may be resolved. For instance, in the case of representing credentials, either the individual has the degree or certificate or has met the qualifications. In other instances, it is not always clear, as in the case of professional conflicts of interest.

It is with utmost importance that the professions of speech-language pathology and audiology continue to monitor and "police" themselves. If an ethical dilemma is not resolved through an informal conversation between professionals, then the individual must be reported to the proper board or agency (AAA, 2006; ASHA, 2004g).

References

American Academy of Audiology. (2003). Code of ethics of the American Academy of Audiology. Retrieved May 19, 2006, from http://www.audiology.org.

American Academy of Audiology. (2004a). Buying groups, rewards, and conflict of interest. *Audiology Today, 16*(3), 38.

American Academy of Audiology. (2004b). Buying groups, trips, cash rebates and conflicts of interest. *Audiology Today, 16*(1), 9.

American Academy of Audiology. (2004c). Guidelines for ethical practice in research for audiologists. *Audiology Today, 15*(6), 14–17.

American Academy of Audiology. (2005). *Ethics in audiology: Guidelines for ethical conduct in clinical, educational, and research settings.* Retrieved May 19, 2006, from http://www.audiology.org.

American Speech-Language-Hearing Association. (1991). Business, marketing, ethics, and professionalism in audiology: An updated annotated bibliography (1986–1989). *ASHA, 33* (Suppl. 3), 39–45.

American Speech-Language-Hearing Association. (1993). *Model Bill of Rights for people receiving audiology or speech-language pathology services.* Retrieved May 19, 2006, from http://www.asha.org.

American Speech-Language-Hearing Association. (1996). Guidelines on the audiologist's role in occupational and environmental hearing conservation. *ASHA, 38* (Suppl. 16), 34–41.

American Speech-Language-Hearing Association. (2001). *Scope of practice in speech language pathology.* Rockville, MD: Author.

American Speech-Language-Hearing Association. (2002a). *Definition of ASHA's continuing education units.* Retrieved May 19, 2006, from http://www.asha.org.

American Speech-Language-Hearing Association. (2002b). Drawing cases for private practice from primary place of employment. *ASHA Supplement, 22,* 225–226.

American Speech-Language-Hearing Association. (2002c). Ethics in research and professional practice. *ASHA Supplement, 22,* 219–221.

American Speech-Language-Hearing Association. (2002d). Knowledge and skills needed by speech-language pathologists providing services to individuals with swallowing and/or feeding disorders. *ASHA Supplement, 22,* 81–88.

American Speech-Language-Hearing Association. (2002e). Public announcements and public statements. *ASHA Supplement, 22,* 223.

American Speech-Language-Hearing Association. (2002f). Rights and responsibilities of test takers: Guidelines and expectations. *ASHA Desk Reference,* Vol. 1, 305–311.

American Speech-Language-Hearing Association. (2003). Code of ethics. *ASHA Supplement, 22,* 13–15.

American Speech-Language-Hearing Association. (2004a). Clinical practice by certificate holders in the profession in which they are not certified. *ASHA Supplement, 24,* 39–40.

American Speech-Language-Hearing Association. (2004b). Competition. *ASHA Supplement, 24,* 41–42.

American Speech-Language-Hearing Association. (2004c). Conflicts of professional interest. *ASHA Supplement, 24,* 46–48.

American Speech-Language-Hearing Association. (2004d). *Evidence-based practice in communication disorders: An introduction* [Technical report]. Retrieved May 19, 2006, from http://www. asha.org.

American Speech-Language-Hearing Association. (2004e). Representation of services for insurance reimbursement or funding. *ASHA Supplement, 24,* 1–3.

American Speech-Language-Hearing Association. (2004f). Scope of practice in audiology. *ASHA Supplement, 24,* 1–9.

American Speech-Language-Hearing Association. (2004g). *Statement of practices and procedures of the Board of Ethics.* Retrieved May 19, 2006, from http:// www.asha.org.

American Speech-Language-Hearing Association. (2004h). Technical report: Cochlear implants. *ASHA Supplement, 24,* 1–35.

American Speech-Language-Hearing Association. (2005a). Knowledge and skills needed by speech-language pathologists providing services to individuals with cognitive communication disorders. *ASHA Supplement,* 1–7.

American Speech-Language-Hearing Association. (2005b). *Protection of human subjects* [Issues in Ethics]. Retrieved May 19, 2006, from http://www.asha.org.

American Speech-Language-Hearing Association. (2005c). *Quality indicators for professional service programs in audiology and speech-language pathology.* Retrieved May 19, 2006, from http://www.asha.org.

National Council of State Board of Examiners for Speech-Language Pathology and Audiology (NCSB). (2006). List of state board Web sites. Retrieved May 19, 2006, from http://www.ncsb.net.

Chapter 8

Professionalism

Learning Objectives
After reading this chapter, you should be able to:

- Operationally define professionalism.
- Recognize unprofessional conduct.
- Apply ethical principles to resolving unprofessional conduct.

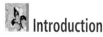 Introduction

Speech-language pathologists (SLPs) and audiologists (AUDs) are aware of their responsibilities to the professions and to those with whom they work: students, clients, supervisors, and other professionals. It is recognized that speech-language pathology and audiology are autonomous professions, that is, self-governing or functionally independent. These professionals must ensure that anyone under their supervision does not engage in any practice that is an ethical violation. Unprofessional activities are prohibited: dishonesty, fraud, deceit, misrepresentation, and sexual harassment.

Speech-language pathologists and audiologists respect individual differences, including those based on race, ethnicity, gender, age, religion, national origin, sexual orientation, and disability. They uphold research standards related to authorship and referencing of others' work or data.

When speech-language-hearing professionals believe that there may have been an ethical violation, an effort should be made for informal resolution. If not resolved informally, ethical violations should be reported to the appropriate boards of ethics. Speech-language pathologists and audiologists need to cooperate with investigations being conducted by the board. Failure to report an ethics violation and failure to cooperate in an ethics investigation are themselves ethics violations. Each of the ethical codes (ASHA, 2003; AAA, 2003a) describes professional responsibilities. These responsibilities include maintaining professional standards, appropriate publication practices, reporting ethical violations, cooperating with ethics boards, and avoiding sexual harassment and unfair discrimination A comparison of these principles and rules is presented in Table 8-1.

This chapter presents a number of case scenarios related to professionalism. The following sections provide scenarios that illustrate several of the principles and rules of the codes of ethics of ASHA and/or AAA. General focus

Table 8-1 Principles and Rules Related to Professionalism in the ASHA
(2003) and AAA (2003a) Codes of Ethics

AAA	Operational Definition	ASHA
1, 8	Professional standards	IV
3a	Prohibit ethical violations	IV-A
8b	Unprofessional behavior	IV-B
2c	Sexual harassment	IV-C
7a	Publication credit	IV-D
7a	Reference citations	IV-E
7b	Accurate description of professional activities	IV-F
—	Autonomy	IV-G
1b	Unfair discrimination	IV-H
8c	Reporting ethical violations	IV-I
8a	Cooperate with ethics board	IV-J

questions need to be asked in order to make decisions about cases. These include the following questions:

1. What information is needed to identify and delineate the problem?
2. What are the possible courses of action?
3. Is there a need for consultation? If so, what type of consultation?
4. How will the plan of action be implemented and monitored?

Prohibiting Ethical Violations

Speech-language-hearing professionals with the CCC and/or members of AAA shall prohibit anyone under their supervision from engaging in any practice that violates the Code of Ethics. Students, speech-language pathology assistants, and professionals in other disciplines may be required by their supervisor to engage in various activities that might violate this ethical rule. Although students, SLP assistants, or other professionals are often exempt from upholding the ASHA and AAA codes of ethics, it is important to discuss how these situations are identified and resolved.

SCENARIO 8-1

An SLP who holds the CCC is supervising graduate students from a local university. During the internship, a graduate student is asked by the supervisor to do a diagnostic evaluation without having previously consulted about the case; no supervision is provided during the evaluation.

Points to Consider

1. What should the student do?
2. What should the university do?
3. What if the supervisor denies that this happened and that the student misunderstood what was to be done?

Suggestions

1. Review the document *Supervision of Student Clinicians* (ASHA, 1994).
2. Discuss the situation with the university supervisor prior to discussing anything with the on-site practicum supervisor. Review procedures for documentation of ethical violations at http://www.asha.org.
3. Review the use of support personnel (ASHA, 2004g).
4. Consult state licensure law and code of conduct for employees at the work setting.

SCENARIO 8-2

An AUD supervising graduate students encourages her students to routinely bill for tympanometry and add an additional charge for acoustic reflexes.

Points to Consider

1. Because obtaining acoustic reflex thresholds is standard for an audiometric battery, does this constitute "padding" the bill?
2. Is this an appropriate activity to teach students?
3. Who should the student consult?

Suggestions

1. Review the preferred practice patterns for audiology (ASHA, 1997).
2. Review *Model Bill of Rights for People Receiving Audiology or Speech-Language Pathology Services* (ASHA, 1993).

Unprofessional Behavior

Both ASHA and AAA have rules that prohibit their members from engaging in dishonesty, fraud, deceit, misrepresentation, sexual harassment, or any other form of conduct that adversely reflects on the professions or on an individual's fitness to serve persons professionally. Furthermore, professionals shall not engage in sexual activities with clients or students over whom they exercise professional authority.

Scenario 8-3

An ASHA-certified SLP provides treatment for an adult male with a fluency disorder. The client asks the clinician to go on a date.

Points to Consider

1. Should the clinician accept?
2. What if the relationship becomes more serious?
3. Who should the SLP consult about this?

Suggestions

1. Review *Model Bill of Rights for People Receiving Audiology or Speech-Language Pathology Services* (ASHA, 1993).
2. Review the code of conduct from the clinician's place of employment regarding personal relationships with clients and discuss this with the supervisor.

Scenario 8-4

An AUD providing hearing aid maintenance through a home health program inappropriately touches some of his female clients when he is in their homes.

Points to Consider

1. Can disciplinary action be sought through the licensing board?
2. In this kind of situation with only two people present, how might the AUD protect his reputation?

Suggestions

1. For Question 1 in Points to Consider, have the clients report this to the AUD's immediate supervisor or the local Council on Aging.
2. For Question 2, review state licensing board guidelines for reporting ethical violations and jurisdictions of ASHA (ASHA, 2002a).
3. For Question 3, consult the procedures utilized by the employer when making home visits. If not addressed, then ask the supervisor to develop procedures.
4. Review the procedures and principles for protection of human subjects (ASHA, 2005b).

Publication Credit

Speech-language pathologists, audiologists, and speech-language-hearing scientists engage in various types of research that may lead to publication. The professionals shall assign credit only to those who have contributed to a publication, presentation, or product. It is important that credit be assigned in proportion to the contribution and only with the contributor's consent. The amount of contribution made by a professional should be discussed with all authors and suggestions made as to how credit will be recognized.

SCENARIO 8-5

A professor who holds the CCC-SLP has been the major advisor for a doctoral student. The results from the dissertation are submitted to a referred journal, but the professor asks the student to list him as first author.

Points to Consider

1. Is this an ethical dilemma?
2. Could a compromise be reached between the professor and the doctoral student?

Suggestions

1. Review the issues in ethics and professional practice (ASHA, 2002b).

2. Discuss the procedure for assigning the order of authorship utilizing the *Publication Manual of the American Psychological Association* ([APA], 2001) and the APA *Ethical Principles of Psychologists and Code of Conduct* (APA, 2002).
3. Determine if the university or department has a procedure or policy for assigning the order of authorship.

SCENARIO 8-6

A physician participates in a research project with two AUDs with CCC-AUD and membership in AAA on migraine headaches that are associated with dizziness. The physician provides diagnosis, patient management, and treatment data. The physician does not do any writing but insists on being the first author.

Points to Consider

1. Is it ethical for the AUDs who planned the project and wrote the paper to list the physician first?
2. Can this ethical rule from ASHA and/or AAA help the AUD in handling the situation with the physician? If so, how?
3. If not listed as first author, how might the physician be listed?

Suggestions

1. Have the AUD share with the physician a copy of the AAA (2003a) and ASHA (2003) codes of ethics.
2. Review any policies or procedures that the work setting may have regarding the assignment of credit for publication.
3. Ask other colleagues at http://www.aaa.org and http://www.asha.org under "discussion forums" to determine policies and procedures that may exist in other work settings.

Reference Citations

Speech-language-hearing professionals and scientists engage in research and utilize resources from various disciplines and other professions. The ASHA-certified clinicians and AAA members shall reference the source when using other persons' ideas, research, presentations, or products in written, oral, or any other media presentation or summary.

SCENARIO 8-7

An SLP with a CCC is providing a workshop to a group of professionals about language/literacy development in children. The SLP provides treatment strategies but does not reference the source(s) because several strategies have been slightly changed.

Points to Consider

1. Why may this be an ethical issue?
2. What should a participant at the workshop do who knows that references have not been given credit or cited?

Suggestions

1. Review the role of ethics in research and professional practice (ASHA, 2002b).
2. Review the definitions of **plagiarism** and **"lazy writing"** (see Glossary) and guidelines regarding plagiarism with the presenter (APA, 2001).

SCENARIO 8-8

An AUD delivers a lecture on current trends in audiology to a group of ENT physicians in his area. He failed to include the source of the information presented in the lecture.

Points to Consider

1. Should he be held ethically liable for not reporting this information?
2. How can sources be recognized in an oral presentation?

Suggestions

1. Share with the AUD the codes of ethics for professional organizations regarding the use of referencing sources (ASHA, 2003; AAA, 2003a).
2. Have the AUD prepare a list of sources that were used for the oral presentation and distribute to the participants.

Reporting Results

All statements to colleagues about professional services, research results, and products shall adhere to prevailing professional standards and shall contain no misrepresentations. It is important that speech-language-hearing professionals be certain about the accuracy of information that is disseminated to the public.

SCENARIO 8-9

A certified SLP provides a wide range of services in a private practice. The SLP has attended several workshops about dyslexia and is described in the brochure about the practice as a "fully certified diagnostician for dyslexia."

Points to Consider

1. Why may this practice involve misrepresentation?
2. What do you think the prevailing professional standard is?

Suggestions

1. Review guidelines for public announcements and statements (ASHA, 2002c).
2. Consult the state licensing board rules and regulations regarding public statements. See National Council of State Board of Examiners for Speech-Language Pathology and Audiology at http://www.ncsb.net (NCSB, 2006).

SCENARIO 8-10

An AUD, a member of AAA and ASHA, is employed by a hearing aid company to market new products. Her sales pitch to dispensing AUDs boasts that her company's new line of products not only has been "clinically" proven to reduce background noise but also provides all clients with significantly enhanced aided speech discrimination scores. Clinical trials of the products have proven that the hearing aids are performing well but not at the level she is claiming.

Points to Consider

1. Is she violating the codes of ethics by providing AUDs with misleading information about the product?
2. What kinds of situations could pressure an AUD in this position to make unwarranted claims?
3. How could this kind of pressure be handled or avoided?

Suggestions

1. Review the AAA Code of Ethics (2003a) regarding use of research.
2. Review and discuss the paper *Evidence-Based Practice in Communication Disorders* (ASHA, 2004c).
3. Consult the code of business conduct for the company regarding Institutional Review Board procedures.
4. Review guidelines for research regarding hearing aids of the Food and Drug Administration (2006) Web site http://www.fda.gov.

Autonomy

Speech-language pathologists and audiologists regard themselves as professionals who make independent judgments about client services everyday. The principle of **autonomy** indicates that the judgments being made are independent of referral source or prescription.

SCENARIO 8-11

An SLP with a CCC enters into a cooperative agreement with a pediatrician that all children seen by the pediatrician will be referred to the SLP. The SLP realizes it is important to have physician referral for reimbursement.

Points to Consider

1. How may this be an ethical dilemma?
2. What are some alternatives for the SLP?

Suggestion

1. Review the papers *Competition* (ASHA, 2004a) and *Preferred Practice Patterns for the Profession of Speech-Language Pathology* (2004d).

SCENARIO 8-12

An ENT physician referring clients for amplification has a habit of recommending specific hearing aids. Although the AUD often disagrees with the physician's recommendations, she fits clients based on his recommendations, ignoring her own professional judgment.

Points to Consider

1. Should she continue to practice with this physician under these circumstances?
2. How could she handle this situation with the physician? With her client?

Suggestions

1. Review the paper *Prescription* (ASHA, 2001a) and the guidelines *Preferred Practice Patterns for the Profession of Audiology* (ASHA, 1996).
2. Review the book *Ethics in Audiology: Guidelines for Ethical Conduct in Clinical, Educational, and Research Settings* (AAA, 2006).

Nondiscrimination

Discrimination must be avoided. Speech-language-hearing professionals must ensure that their relationships with colleagues, students, and members of allied professions are not based on race or ethnicity, gender, age, religion, national origin, sexual orientation, or disability.

SCENARIO 8-13

An SLP with a CCC from ASHA works with a licensed physical therapist (PT) who is a native of Iran. The SLP mentions to a client that the PT was recently interviewed by the FBI. The client tells the PT that he is discontinuing services because of a connection with terrorists.

Point to Consider

1. Has an ethical violation by the SLP occurred?

Suggestions

1. Review the papers *Confidentiality* (ASHA, 2004b) and "Cultural Competence" (ASHA, 2005a).
2. Discuss the code of conduct at the business regarding working relationships with other allied health professionals.

SCENARIO 8-14

Mrs. Collins, a pediatric AUD, refuses to refer children for speech-language evaluations to Mrs. Martinez, a competent SLP in her town. Although Mrs. Martinez is well qualified with children, Mrs. Collins would rather not refer a Caucasian child to a Hispanic clinician.

Points to Consider

1. Is Mrs. Martinez being discriminated against?
2. Are there situations in which Mrs. Martinez could have difficulty with a child of different ethnicity?
3. Who should decide if this is an ethical dilemma?
4. Is Mrs. Collins considering individual issues and needs or acting on a bias?

Suggestions

1. Review the paper *Cultural Competence* (ASHA, 2005a).
2. Review the book *Ethics in Audiology: Guidelines for Ethical Conduct in Clinical, Educational, and Research Settings* (AAA, 2006).

3. Discuss the position statement regarding students and professionals who speak English with accents and nonstandard dialects (ASHA Joint Subcommittee of the Executive Board on English Language Proficiency, 1998).

Reporting Ethical Violations

If a member of AAA and ASHA witnesses a violation of either code of ethics, there are several options. As discussed previously, this ethical dilemma may be handled directly with the professional and possibly be resolved. If there is reason to believe that either code of ethics has been violated and no resolution is achieved, then the individual shall inform the ethics board.

SCENARIO 8-15

An SLP-CF tells another SLP who holds the CCC that the supervisor at work is possibly committing fraudulent billing.

Points to Consider

1. How should the clinicians proceed?
2. Should a process of ethical decision making be followed?

Suggestions

1. Discuss the paper *Representation of Services for Insurance Reimbursement or Funding* (ASHA, 2004e).
2. Review the *Statement of Practices and Procedures of the Board of Ethics* (ASHA, 2004f).

SCENARIO 8-16

An AUD with a CCC has become aware that his business partner is committing Medicaid fraud with his billing practices.

Point to Consider

1. Could this AUD be held responsible for the violation of ethics of his business partner if he does not report it?

Suggestions

1. Review the same documents reviewed in Scenario 8-15.
2. Review procedures for reporting ethical violations with the state Medicaid office (Centers for Medicare and Medicaid Services, 2006).
3. Review the book *Ethics in Audiology: Guidelines for Ethical Conduct in Clinical, Educational, and Research Settings* (AAA, 2006).

Cooperating with the Ethics Boards

Cooperating with the ethics boards for ASHA and AAA is an important part of the process of an investigation by a board. It involves full disclosure and being honest and truthful with the board.

SCENARIO 8-17

A certified SLP reports an ethical violation to ASHA's Board of Ethics but does not want to provide any personal identification to the board.

Point to Consider

1. Can anonymous reports of a suspected ethical violation be done? Why or why not?

Suggestion

1. Review the *Statement of Practices and Procedures of the Board of Ethics* (ASHA, 2004f).

SCENARIO 8-18

Mr. Smith, an AUD in private practice, was recently found in violation of several codes of ethics by ASHA's Board of

Ethics. In addition, the state licensing board took disciplinary action. He is planning to sue the state's licensing board over the choice of disciplinary action taken against him.

Points to Consider

1. Is Mr. Smith correct in seeking legal action against the licensing board?
2. Does this ethical proscription obligate Mr. Smith to the state licensing board or to ASHA?
3. Was AAA's Ethical Practices Board notified?

Suggestions

1. Review *Rules and Procedures for Appeals* (ASHA, 2001b).
2. Consult the state licensing board rules and regulations regarding use of public statements (NCSB, 2006).

Summary

Professionalism encompasses a variety of areas for SLPs and AUDs. It is important to have an amenable working relationship with others and maintain high standards of professional behavior. Public trust and respect from other professionals must be developed and maintained. Sexual harassment results in diminished respect for the professional if alleged and the professional is found guilty.

It is important to guard against any type of behavior that may be considered as unprofessional. In addition, giving proper credit for publication and citing references for others' work have important legal implications. These practices are done to avoid plagiarism and copyright violations. Professional organizations and associations, licensing boards, state speech-language-hearing associations, and businesses have little tolerance for unprofessional behavior. If violations are not resolved with other colleagues, then it is the responsibility of the professional to report the alleged violation and fully cooperate with the ethics board and/or professional organization that may need to impose sanctions.

References

American Academy of Audiology (AAA). (2003a). *Code of ethics of the American Academy of Audiology.* Retrieved May 19, 2006, from http://www.audiology.org.

American Academy of Audiology. (2003b). *Guidelines for ethical practice in research for audiologists.* Retrieved May 19, 2006, from http://www.audiology.org.

American Academy of Audiology. (2005). *Ethics in audiology: Guidelines for ethical conduct in clinical, educational, and research settings.* Retrieved May 19, 2006, from http://www.audiology.org.

American Academy of Private Practice in Speech Pathology and Audiology. (2006). *Valuing your business.* Retrieved May 19, 2006, from http://www.aappspa.org.

American Psychological Association (APA). (2001). *Publication manual of the American Psychological Association* (5th ed.). Washington, DC: Author.

American Psychological Association. (2002). *Ethical principles of psychologists and code of conduct.* Retrieved May 19, 2006, from http://www.apa.org.

American Speech-Language-Hearing Association (ASHA). (1993). *Model bill of rights for people receiving audiology or speech-language pathology services.* Retrieved May 19, 2006, from http://www.asha.org.

American Speech-Language-Hearing Association. (1994, March). Supervision of student clinicians. *ASHA, 36* (Suppl. 13), 13–14.

American Speech-Language-Hearing Association. (1997). *Preferred practice patterns for the profession of audiology.* Rockville, MD: Author. Also see http://www.asha.org.

American Speech-Language-Hearing Association. (2001a). Prescription. *ASHA Supplement, 22,* 215–216.

American Speech-Language-Hearing Association. (2001b). *Rules and procedures for appeals.* Retrieved May 19, 2006, from http://www.asha.org.

American Speech-Language-Hearing Association. (2002a). Ethical practice inquiries: ASHA jurisdictions. *ASHA Supplement, 22,* 231–232.

American Speech-Language-Hearing Association. (2002b). Ethics in research and professional practice. *ASHA Supplement, 22,* 219–221.

American Speech-Language-Hearing Association. (2002c). Public announcements and public statements. *ASHA Supplement, 22,* 223.

American Speech-Language-Hearing Association. (2003). Code of ethics. *ASHA Supplement, 22,* 13–15.

American Speech-Language-Hearing Association. (2004a). Competition. *ASHA Supplement, 24,* 41–42.

American Speech-Language-Hearing Association. (2004b). Confidentiality. *ASHA Supplement, 24,* 43–45.

American Speech-Language-Hearing Association. (2004c). *Evidence-based practice in communication disorders: An introduction* [Technical report]. Retrieved from http://www.asha.org.

American Speech-Language-Hearing Association. (2004d). *Preferred practice patterns for the profession of speech-language pathology.* Retrieved May 19, 2006, from http://www.asha.org.

American Speech-Language-Hearing Association. (2004e). Representation of services for insurance reimbursement or funding. *ASHA Supplement, 24,* 1–3.

American Speech-Language-Hearing Association. (2004f). *Statement of practices and procedures of the Board of Ethics.* Retrieved May 19, 2006, from http://www.asha.org.

American Speech-Language-Hearing Association. (2004g). *Support personnel.* Retrieved May 19, 2006, from http://www.asha.org.

American Speech-Language-Hearing Association. (2005a). Cultural competence. *ASHA Supplement, 25,* 1–2.

American Speech-Language-Hearing Association. (2005b). *Protection of human subjects.* [Issues in Ethics]. Retrieved May 19, 2006, from http://www.asha.org.

American Speech-Language-Hearing Association Joint Subcommittee of the Executive Board on English Language Proficiency. (1998). Students and professionals who speak English with accents and nonstandard dialects: Issues and recommendations. Position statement and technical report. *ASHA, 40* (Suppl. 18), 83.

Centers for Medicare and Medicaid Services. (2006). *Fraud and abuse.* Retrieved May 19, 2006, from http://www.cms.hhs.gov.

Food and Drug Administration. (2006). Retrieved May 19, 2006, from http://www.fda.gov.

National Council of State Board of Examiners for Speech-Language Pathology and Audiology. (2006). *List of state board Web sites.* Retrieved May 19, 2006, from http://www.ncsb.net.

Epilogue

In Chapter 1 of the book, professionalism and ethics were defined and discussed. Chapter 2 and Chapter 3 described the evolution of the ASHA and AAA codes of ethics, including selected areas, future issues, and comparison of the codes. Chapter 4 summarized factors that may influence values and beliefs, described a model for ethical decision making, offered suggestions for reporting violations, and described various types of ethics enforcement that may be done. Chapter 5 to Chapter 8 provided an analysis of scenarios that illustrated different principles and rules with related references.

Ethics have always been important to the professionals of speech-language pathology and audiology. Ethical practice is in the best interest of those served (i.e., clients, students, supervisors, colleagues, and other professionals) by speech-language-hearing professionals. During the 1990s, there was an increased level of attention to ethics—most likely as the result of emerging areas of practice and new challenges. ASHA's Code of Ethics was revised five times during the 1990s and once in both 2001 and 2003. The first AAA Code of Ethics was adopted in the fall of 1990, published in 1991, and then later revised. With each of the changes, both ASHA and AAA have developed several other publications through supplements, position statements, technical reports and books. Ethics are dynamic with an endless cycle of change. This means that clinicians must be current about new developments in ethics and must work proactively for ethical practice in professional activities: teaching, service, and research.

Several current issues warrant continued consideration. Among these issues are ethics education, expanded scope of professional practice, and serving the needs of increasingly diverse populations and practice settings. Given the rapidly changing nature of educational health care services, it is likely that many new ethical challenges will emerge in the coming years. Readers of this textbook must continue to discuss and resolve ethical dilemmas as these new areas of practice emerge and develop.

Ethical principles and rules are often interrelated, and it is important to note that one's level of understanding of these principles could impact other areas of practice. Ethical decisions are not made in a "vacuum" and often involve careful analysis and consideration from several points of view. Any speech-language-hearing professional making ethical decisions must be mindful that the potential impact of each ethical decision could influence outcomes.

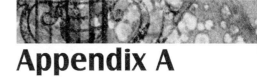

Appendix A

American Speech-Language-Hearing Association Code of Ethics (2003)

Operational Classification of ASHA's Code of Ethics	
	Competence
	Referral
	Avoid Prejudice or Partiality
	Fidelity: honesty
	Delegation of duties
	Full disclosure
Beneficence; doing good	Effectiveness of services and products
	Avoiding guarantees
	Correspondence
	Telecommunication
	Documentation
	Confidentiality; information disclosure
	Fraud
	Informed consent
	Substance abuse
	ASHA's CCC
	Scope of competence

Operational Classification of ASHA's Code of Ethics (*Continued*)	
Competence	Continuing education
	Delegating duties
	Scope of competence
	Maintenance of equipment
	Accurate representation of credentials
	Conflict of interest
	Financial conflict of interest
Public statements	Accurate documentation
	Accurate information
	Uphold professional standards
	Prohibit ethical violations
	Avoid unprofessional behavior
Professionalism	Sexual misconduct
	Publication credit
	Reference citations
	Clinical and research reports
	Autonomy
	Justice; fair allocation
	Reporting ethical violations
	Cooperating with Board of Ethics

Preamble

The preservation of the highest standards of integrity and ethical principles is vital to the responsible discharge of obligations by speech-language pathologists; audiologists; and speech, language, and hearing scientists. This Code of Ethics sets forth the fundamental principles and rules considered essential to this purpose.

Every individual who is (1) a member of the American Speech-Language-Hearing Association, whether certified or not, (2) a nonmember holding the Certificate of Clinical Competence from the association, (3) an applicant for membership or certification, or (4) a clinical fellow seeking to fulfill standards for certification shall abide by this Code of Ethics.

Any violation of the spirit and purpose of this Code shall be considered unethical. Failure to specify any particular responsibility or practice in this Code of Ethics shall not be construed as denial of the existence of such responsibilities or practices.

The fundamentals of ethical conduct are described by Principles of Ethics and by Rules of Ethics as they relate to the conduct of research and scholarly activities and responsibility to persons served; the public; and speech-language pathologists, audiologists, and speech, language, and hearing scientists.

Principles of Ethics, aspirational and inspirational in nature, form the underlying moral basis for the Code of Ethics. Individuals shall observe these principles as affirmative obligations under all conditions of professional activity. Rules of Ethics are specific statements of minimally acceptable professional conduct or of prohibitions and are applicable to all individuals.

Principle of Ethics I

Individuals shall honor their responsibilities to hold paramount the welfare of persons they serve professionally or participants in research and scholarly activities and shall treat animals involved in research in a humane manner.

Rules of Ethics

A. Individuals shall provide all services competently.
B. Individuals shall use every resource, including referral when appropriate, to ensure that high-quality service is provided.
C. Individuals shall not discriminate in the delivery of professional services or the conduct of research and

scholarly activities on the basis of race or ethnicity, gender, age, religion, national origin, sexual orientation, or disability.

D. Individuals shall not misrepresent the credentials of assistants, technicians, support personnel and shall inform those they serve professionally of the name and professional credentials of persons providing services.

E. Individuals who hold the Certificate of Clinical Competency shall not delegate tasks that require the unique skills, knowledge, and judgment that are within the scope of their profession to assistants, technicians, support personnel, students, or any nonprofessionals over whom they have supervisory responsibility. An individual may delegate support services to assistants, technicians, support personnel, students, or any other persons only if those services are adequately supervised by an individual who holds the appropriate Certificate of Clinical Competence.

F. Individuals shall fully inform the persons they serve of the nature and possible effects of services rendered and products dispensed, and they shall inform participants in research about the possible effects of their participation in research conducted.

G. Individuals shall evaluate the effectiveness of services rendered and of products dispensed and shall provide services or dispense products only when benefit can reasonably be expected.

H. Individuals shall not guarantee the results of any treatment or procedure, directly or by implication; however, they may make a reasonable statement of prognosis.

I. Individuals shall not provide clinical services solely by correspondence.

J. Individuals may practice by telecommunication (for example, telehealth/e-health) where not prohibited by law.

K. Individuals shall adequately maintain and appropriately secure records of professional services rendered, research and scholarly activities conducted, and products dispensed and shall allow access to these records only when authorized or when required by law.

L. Individuals shall not reveal, without authorization, any professional or personal information about identified persons served professionally or identified participants involved in research and scholarly activities unless required by law to do so, or unless doing so is necessary to protect the welfare of the person or of the community or otherwise required by law.

M. Individuals shall not charge for services not rendered, nor shall they misrepresent services rendered, products dispensed, or research and scholarly activities conducted.

N. Individuals shall use persons in research or as subjects of teaching demonstrations only with their informed consent.

O. Individuals whose professional services are adversely affected by substance abuse or other health-related conditions shall seek professional assistance and, where appropriate, withdraw from the affected areas of practice.

Principle of Ethics II

Individuals shall honor their responsibility to achieve and maintain the highest level of professional competence.

Rules of Ethics

A. Individuals shall engage in the provision of clinical services only when they hold the appropriate Certificate of Clinical Competence or when they are in the certification process and are supervised by an individual who holds the appropriate Certificate of Clinical Competence.

B. Individuals shall engage in only those aspects of the professions that are within the scope of their competence, considering their level of education, training, and experience.

C. Individuals shall continue their professional development throughout their careers.

D. Individuals shall delegate the provision of clinical services only to: (1) persons who hold the appropriate Certificate of Clinical Competence; (2) persons in the education or certification process who are appropriately supervised by an individual who holds the appropriate Certificate of Clinical Competence; or (3) assistants, technicians, or support personnel who are adequately supervised by an individual who holds the appropriate Certificate of Clinical Competence.

E. Individuals shall not require or permit their professional staff to provide services or conduct research activities that exceed the staff members' competence, level of education, training, and experience.

F. Individuals shall ensure that all equipment used in the provision of services or to conduct research and scholarly activities is in proper working order and is properly calibrated.

Principle of Ethics III

Individuals shall honor their responsibility to the public by promoting public understanding of the professions; by supporting the development of services designed to fulfill the unmet needs of the public; and by providing accurate information in all communications involving any aspect of the professions, including dissemination of research findings and scholarly activities.

Rules of Ethics

A. Individuals shall not misrepresent their credentials, competence, education, training, experience, or scholarly or research contributions.

B. Individuals shall not participate in professional activities that constitute a conflict of interest.

C. Individuals shall refer those served professionally solely on the basis of the interest of those being referred and not on any personal financial interest.

D. Individuals shall not misrepresent diagnostic information, research, services rendered, or products dispensed; neither shall they engage in any scheme to defraud in connection with obtaining payment or reimbursement for such services or products.

E. Individuals' statements to the public shall provide accurate information about the nature and management of communication disorders, about the professions, about professional services, and about research and scholarly activities.

F. Individuals' statements to the public—advertising, announcing, and marketing their professional services; reporting research results; and promoting products—shall adhere to prevailing professional standards and shall not contain misrepresentations.

Principle of Ethics IV

Individuals shall honor their responsibilities to the professions and their relationships with colleagues, students, and members of allied professions. Individuals shall uphold the dignity and autonomy of the professions, maintain harmonious interprofessional and intraprofessional relationships, and accept the professions' self-imposed standards.

Rules of Ethics

A. Individuals shall prohibit anyone under their supervision from engaging in any practice that violates the Code of Ethics.

B. Individuals shall not engage in dishonesty, fraud, deceit, misrepresentation, sexual harassment, or any other form of conduct that adversely reflects on the professions or on the individuals' fitness to serve persons professionally.

C. Individuals shall not engage in sexual activities with clients or students over whom they exercise professional authority.

D. Individuals shall assign credit only to those who contributed to a publication, presentation, or product.

Credit shall be assigned in proportion to the contribution and only with the contributor's consent.

E. Individuals shall reference the source when using other persons' ideas, research, presentations, or products in written, oral, or any other media presentation or summary.

F. Individuals' statements to colleagues about professional services, research results, and products shall adhere to prevailing professional standards and shall contain no misrepresentations.

G. Individuals shall not provide professional services without exercising independent professional judgment, regardless of referral source or prescription.

H. Individuals shall not discriminate in their relationships with colleagues, students, and members of allied professions on the basis of race or ethnicity, gender, age, religion, national origin, sexual orientation, or disability.

I. Individuals who have reason to believe that the Code of Ethics has been violated shall inform the Board of Ethics.

J. Individuals shall comply fully with the policies of the Board of Ethics in its consideration and adjudication of violations of the Code of Ethics.

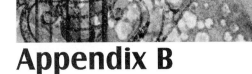

Appendix B

American Academy of Audiology
Code of Ethics (2003)*

Operational Classification of AAA's Code of Ethics	
Honesty and compassion	Justice and fidelity
Competence	Education and experience
	Referrals
	Avoid harm
	Discrimination
	Supervision and delegation
	Prohibit ethical violations
	Maintain competence
Confidentiality	Consent
Best interest of persons served	Avoid exploitation
	Accurate charge for services
	Avoid conflict of interest
	Informed consent

*Note. Courtesy of the American Academy of Audiology.

Operational Classification of AAA's Code of Ethics (*Continued*)	
Accurate information	Information about services and products
	Accurate prognosis
	Product-oriented research
	Privacy and informed consent
	Documentation
Professionalism	Accurate representation: education, training, credentials, competence
	Public statements: services, products, research
Public and professional responsibilities	Conflict of interest
	Maintain professional standards of reporting products and services
Ethical conduct	Comply with Code of Ethics
	Avoid dishonesty: illegal conduct
	Report ethical violations
	Cooperate with Ethical Practices Board

Preamble

The Code of Ethics of the American Academy of Audiology specifies professional standards that allow for the proper discharge of audiologists' responsibilities to those served and that protect the integrity of the profession. The Code of Ethics consists of two parts. The first part, the Statement of Principles and Rules, presents precepts that members of the Academy agree to uphold. The second part, the Procedures, provides the process that enables enforcement of the Principles and Rules.

Part I: Statement of Principles and Rules

PRINCIPLE 1: Members shall provide professional services and conduct research with honesty and compassion and shall respect the dignity, worth, and rights of those served.

Rule 1a: Individuals shall not limit the delivery of professional services on any basis that is unjustifiable or irrelevant to the need for the potential benefit from such services.

Rule 1b: Individuals shall not provide services except in a professional relationship and shall not discriminate in the provision of services to individuals on the basis of sex, race, religion, national origin, sexual orientation, or general health.

PRINCIPLE 2: Members shall maintain high standards of professional competence in rendering services.

Rule 2a: Members shall provide only those professional services for which they are qualified by education and experience.

Rule 2b: Individuals shall use available resources, including referrals to other specialists, and shall not accept benefits or items of personal value for receiving or making referrals.

Rule 2c: Individuals shall exercise all reasonable precautions to avoid injury to persons in the delivery of professional services or execution of research.

Rule 2d: Individuals shall provide appropriate supervision and assume full responsibility for services delegated to supportive personnel. Individuals shall not delegate any service requiring professional competence to unqualified persons.

Rule 2e: Individuals shall not permit personnel to engage in any practice that is a violation of the Code of Ethics.

Rule 2f: Individuals shall maintain professional competence, including participation in continuing education.

PRINCIPLE 3: Members shall maintain the confidentiality of the information and records of those receiving services or involved in research.

Rule 3a: Individuals shall not reveal to unauthorized persons any professional or personal information obtained from the person served professionally, unless required by law.

PRINCIPLE 4: Members shall provide only services and products that are in the best interest of those served.

Rule 4a: Individuals shall not exploit persons in the delivery of professional services.

Rule 4b: Individuals shall not charge for services not rendered.

Rule 4c: Individuals shall not participate in activities that constitute a conflict of professional interest.

Rule 4d: Individuals using investigational procedures with patients, or prospectively collecting research data, shall first obtain full informed consent from the patient or guardian.

PRINCIPLE 5: Members shall provide accurate information about the nature and management of communicative disorders and about the services and products offered.

Rule 5a: Individuals shall provide persons served with the information a reasonable person would want to know about the nature and possible effects of services rendered, or products provided, or research being conducted.

Rule 5b: Individuals may make a statement of prognosis but shall not guarantee results, mislead, or misinform persons served or studied.

Rule 5c: Individuals shall conduct and report product-related research only according to accepted standards of research practice.

Rule 5d: Individuals shall not carry out teaching or research consent activities in a manner that constitutes an invasion of privacy or that fails to inform persons fully about the nature and possible effects of these activities, affording all persons informed free choice of participation.

Rule 5e: Individuals shall maintain documentation of professional services rendered.

PRINCIPLE 6: Members shall comply with the ethical standards of the Academy with regard to public statements or publication.

Rule 6a: Individuals shall not misrepresent their educational degrees, training, credentials, or competence. Only degrees earned from regionally accredited institutions in which training was obtained in audiology or a directly related discipline may be used in public statements concerning professional services.

Rule 6b: Individuals' public statements about professional services, products, or research results shall not contain representations or claims that are false, misleading, or deceptive.

PRINCIPLE 7: Members shall honor their responsibilities to the public and to professional colleagues.

Rule 7a: Individuals shall not use professional or commercial affiliations in any way that would limit services to or mislead patients or colleagues.

Rule 7b: Individuals shall inform colleagues and the public in a manner consistent with the highest professional standards about products and services they have developed or research they have conducted.

PRINCIPLE 8: Members shall uphold the dignity of the profession and freely accept the Academy's self-imposed standards.

Rule 8a: Individuals shall not violate these Principles and Rules, nor attempt to circumvent them.

Rule 8b: Individuals shall not engage in dishonesty or illegal conduct that adversely reflects on the profession.

Rule 8c: Individuals shall inform the Ethical Practices Board when there are reasons to believe that a member of the Academy may have violated the Code of Ethics.

Rule 8d: Individuals shall cooperate with the Ethical Practices Board in any matter related to the Code of Ethics.

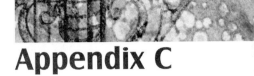

Appendix C

Cross-Index of Ethical Case Scenarios/Scenarios

Many of the scenarios in this book involve issues beyond the subject heading of the section in which the scenario is found. For that reason, the scenarios have been cross-referenced to other topics in the book to which they might also be relevant. The scenarios are indexed by chapter and scenario number. Readers may want to examine the entire set of scenarios as being possibly relevant to that topic.

Topic	Scenario
Audiology	1-1
	4-2
	4-4
	4-7
	5-2
	5-4
	5-6
	5-8
	5-10
	5-12
	5-14
	5-16
	5-18
	5-20
	5-22

188   Appendix C

Topic	Scenario
	6-7
	6-13
	7-10
	8-4
	8-14
Business practices	4-2
	4-3
	4-4
	4-5
	4-6
	5-20
	5-27
	5-28
	6-13
	7-4
	7-6
	7-7
	7-8
	8-2
	8-10
	8-11
	8-12
	8-15
	8-16
Clinical fellowship year (CFY)	4-3
	6-9
Certification	1-1
	5-2
	6-3
	6-4
	6-8
	6-9

Topic	Scenario
	6-12
	7-1
	7-2
	7-11
	8-9
Client/family education	5-6
	5-15
Clinical practice	4-1
	5-2
	5-14
	5-22
	8-1
Competence	1-1
	4-1
	5-2
	5-3
	5-4
	5-5
	5-6
	5-7
	5-8
	5-22
	5-25
	6-1
	6-2
	6-5
	6-7
	6-8
	6-11
	7-2
	7-5
	7-10
	7-11

192   Appendix C

Topic	Scenario
Informed consent	4-4
	5-1
	5-13
	5-14
	5-29
	5-30
	5-31
Institutional Review Board (IRB)	4-4
	5-13
	5-31
	7-9
Licensure	4-5
	5-2
	5-9
	5-11
	6-10
	7-1
	7-7
	7-11
	8-9
	8-18
Maintenance and calibration of equipment	6-13
	6-14
Misrepresentation	5-17
	5-18
	6-9
	6-10
	6-13
	7-1
	7-2

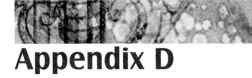

Appendix D

Journals Devoted to Ethics

Bioethics
Biomedical Ethics
Biomedical Ethics Reviews
Cambridge Quarterly of Healthcare Ethics
Clinical Medical Ethics
Ethical Humanist
Ethics
Ethics and Behavior
Ethics and Medicine
Ethics and Policy
Healthcare Ethics
Issues: A Critical Examination of Contemporary Ethical Issues in Health Care
Journal of Clinical Ethics
Journal of Information Ethics
Journal of Law, Medicine, and Ethics
Journal of Mass Media Ethics
Journal of Medical Ethics
Journal of Military Ethics
Journal of Moral Education
Journal of Religious Ethics
Kennedy Institute of Ethics Journal
Legal Ethics

Man and Medicine

Medical Ethics Advisor

Morality

National Reporter on Legal Ethics and Professional Responsibility

New Ethicals Journal

New Titles in Bioethics

Notre Dame Journal of Law, Ethics, and Public Policy

Recent Ethics Opinions

Tanner Lectures on Human Values

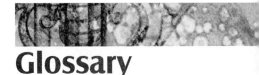

Glossary

abuse Incident or practice that is not consistent with sound professional practices.

allegation Any written or oral statement or other indication of possible ethical misconduct.

alternative dispute resolution A process focusing on alternative ways to resolve disputes, including employers and employees or others in confrontational situations.

anonymity Protection of study participants so that even the investigator cannot identify individuals with the information provided.

arbitrary Subject to individual will or judgment without restriction; capricious.

arbitration Process of resolving conflicts in a structured setting such as formal litigation.

autonomy Freedom of choice, self-determination.

beneficence Fundamental ethical principle that involves doing good for others.

best evidence Selection of studies for inclusion in research reviews only if they are specifically related to the topic, methodologically adequate, and generalizable to a specific situation.

best interest A concept by which the best interests of the individual are considered.

bias Any influence that affects or distorts a decision.

blind review Review of a manuscript or proposal so that neither the author nor the reviewer is identified to the other party.

breach of confidentiality Occurs when someone having access to information shares it with others who have no legitimate reason to know that information.

clinical ethics Ethics that deal with clinical activities and focus on client, clinician, confidentiality, beneficence; structured approach to identifying, analyzing, and resolving ethical issues.

code of conduct Standard of professional conduct.

code of ethics Fundamental ethical principles established by a discipline or institution to guide professional conduct.

competence Ability to provide care according to a standard of care and to the profession's code of ethics.

competency The ability to understand the nature and consequences of the treatment procedure(s).

complainant One who submits a written document describing what may be an ethical violation.

confidentiality Information provided by a client to a

professional will not be revealed to another person.

conflicts of interest   Situations in which personal and/or financial considerations compromise judgment in any professional activity or in which the potential for professional judgment appears to be compromised.

consent   Permit, approve, or comply.

consequentialism   Ethical theory that views the outcome of an action in terms of the consequences of the action.

cybercheating   Internet plagiarism, i.e., copying information directly from the Internet without referencing the source(s).

deontologism   Ethical theory in which some actions are right or wrong for reasons other than their consequences.

descriptive ethics   What people actually believe or how they actually act, regardless of whether their beliefs and actions are justified.

dilemma   Ethical issue or problem.

discrimination   Showing prejudice or partiality; similar to bias.

duplicate submission   Submission of the same manuscript simultaneously to two or more different journals; violation of ethical conduct.

ethical   Evaluation of actions, rules, or character of persons, especially as it refers to rightness or wrongness.

ethical dilemma   Occurs when ethical issues conflict; synonym: *moral dilemma.*

ethical principles   Autonomy; beneficence, nonmaleficence, justice, and professional ethics.

ethics   Generic term for study of rules, principles, and moral values; focuses on what is right or wrong and of what ought to be.

ethics board   Board that deals with ethical problems and dilemmas of professional conduct.

evidence-based practice   Utilization of best available research to make clinical decisions about client care.

fabrication   Fraudulent data, or results.

falsification   Manipulating materials, equipment, or processes or changing or omitting data so that findings are inaccurate.

fidelity   State of being faithful, loyal; keeping promises on agreements.

fraud   Intentional deception or misrepresentation.

gift authorship   Unjustified authorship; including individual as author who did not contribute substantially to a project.

honorary authorship   Unjustified authorship; same as gift authorship.

incompetence   Failure to provide an appropriate level of care and to uphold the code of ethics.

incomplete authorship   Failure to include individuals who contributed substantially to a project; students are most frequently overlooked as authors.

informed consent   Ethical principle that requires obtaining voluntary participation of subjects and clients after informing them of possible risks and benefits.

Institutional Review Board (IRB)   Group of individuals from an institution who meet to review proposed and ongoing research relative to ethical considerations.

irresponsible authorship
Problems related to unjustified authorship, incomplete authorship, and/or inaccurate quotations and/or references.

justice   Fair treatment and allocation of resources; synonym: *moral rightness*.

law   Statutes, rules, and regulations that govern people, relationships, behaviors, and interactions with the state, society, and federal government.

"lazy writing"   Closely related to plagiarism except references are cited; paragraph after paragraph lifted out of one or more sources and presented as a paper.

liability   Responsibility of professional to provide appropriate standard of care or failure to perform a duty that causes harm.

licensure   Legal mechanism by which a government agency authorizes persons who have met minimal standards of competency to engage in a given occupation or profession.

malpractice   Any type of negligence that causes physical or emotional harm.

metaethics   Deals with the nature and meaning of ethical reasons that are valid for judgments about morality.

misrepresentation   Statement by words or other conduct that is likely to mislead, may be intentional or negligent.

moral dilemma   Occurs when moral ideas conflict; synonym: *ethical dilemma*.

morals   Ideas about right and wrong; synonym: *ethics*.

negligence   Failure to use such care as a prudent and careful person would use under similar circumstances; doing some act

that a person of ordinary prudence would not have done under similar circumstances or failure to do what a person of ordinary prudence would have done under similar circumstances. Elements of negligence: duty, breach of duty, proximate cause, and harm or damage.

nonmaleficence   Preventing harm or risk of harm; implies need to be aware of potential risks.

normative ethics   Aimed at identifying, understanding, and applying justified moral views; analysis of values and interests to determine what should be done.

partnership points   Rewards offered by manufacturers to clinicians for dispensing their products which is based on profits and losses.

patchwork plagiarism   Verbatim quote but with some single words changed; references not cited; less severe form of plagiarism.

peer review   Review and evaluation of manuscripts by peers with relevant expertise.

plagiarism   Stealing style, ideas, or phrases. Ranges from word for word (exact) to patchwork (some words changed); sometimes related to incorrect referencing.

practice guidelines   Recommended set of procedures for a specific area of practice, based on research findings and current practice(s).

professional ethics   Ethics to guide professional activities; most professional organizations have a code of ethics.

professional negligence   A negligent act or omission in the delivery of professional services that is the proximate cause of a personal injury or wrongful death, provided that the services are within the scope of services for which the provider is licensed and are within any restriction imposed by the licensing agency or licensed facility.

public health ethics   Ethics that deal with protecting, promoting, and restoring the public's health.

registration   Form of certification administered by a government agency in which persons who have completed required training are listed in a register that is maintained by the agency.

rehabilitation ethics   Moral and ethical concerns that arise during remedial or restorative work with clients, usually in relation to a team of health professionals.

research ethics   Ethics focusing on research; involves ethical conduct of researcher, informed consent, confidentiality.

research misconduct   Fabricating, falsification, or plagiarism or other practices that deviate from professional standards for proposing, conducting, or reporting research.

scope of practice   List of professional activities that define range of services offered within the professions of speech-language pathology and audiology.

standard of care   Level of care that must be provided so as not to be guilty of negligence (malpractice); care that a reasonable and sensible person would provide in the same situation.

telehealth   Providing health care services using interactive video, audio, computer, and advanced telecommunication technologies.

telepractice   Application of telecommunication technology to deliver professional services at a distance. Also known as telehealth or e-health.

unethical   Failure to adhere to ethical guidelines.

unjustified authorship   Authors who did not make substantial contribution(s); synonyms: *gift authorship* and *honorary authorship*.

utilitarianism   Most common form of consequentialism; means that one should act to do greatest good for greatest number; synonym: *social consequentialism*.

virtue   Trait or character that is socially valued.

whistleblower   Person who makes allegations of ethical misconduct.

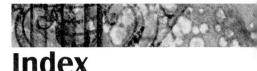

Index

Page numbers followed by the letter "f" indicates figures; "t" indicates tables.